OXFORD MEDICAL PUBLICATIONS

Oncology
A case-based manual

Oncology
A case-based manual

Edited by

Paul R. Harnett

Clinical Associate Professor
University of Sydney and
Director, Department of Medical Oncology and Palliative Care
Westmead Hospital
Sydney

John Cartmill

Senior Lecturer in Surgery
University of Sydney Department of Surgery
Nepean Hospital
Sydney

And

Paul Glare

Clinical Senior Lecturer, University of Sydney and
Head, Palliative Care
Sydney Cancer Centre
Royal Prince Alfred Hospital
Sydney

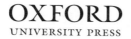

OXFORD
UNIVERSITY PRESS

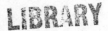
OXFORD

UNIVERSITY PRESS

Great Clarendon Street, Oxford OX2 6DP
Oxford University Press is a department of the University of Oxford.
It furthers the University's objective of excellence in research, scholarship,
and education by publishing worldwide in

Oxford New York
Athens Auckland Bangkok Bogotá Buenos Aires Calcutta
Cape Town Chennai Dar es Salaam Delhi Florence Hong Kong Istanbul
Karachi Kuala Lumpur Madrid Melbourne Mexico City Mumbai
Nairobi Paris São Paulo Singapore Taipei Tokyo Toronto Warsaw
and associated companies in Berlin Ibadan

Oxford is a registered trade mark of Oxford University Press
in the UK and certain other countries

Published in the United States
by Oxford University Press Inc., New York

A catalogue record for this book is available from the British Library

Library of Congress Cataloging in Publication Data
Oncology : a case-based manual / edited by Paul Harnett, John
Cartmill, and Paul Glare.
Includes bibliographical references.
1. Cancer Case studies. I. Harnett, Paul. II. Cartmill, John.
III. Glare, Paul.
[DNLM: 1. Decision Making Case Report. 2. Neoplasms Case Report.
3. Terminal Care Case Report. QZ 200 058206 1999]
RC262.0526   1999   616.99'4—dc21   99–20413

ISBN 0–19–262978–6

Typeset by Footnote Graphics,
Warminster, Wilts
Printed in Great Britain by Bookcraft Ltd., Midsomer Norton, Avon

Contents

Contents

Contents

Preface

This book evolved from our experience teaching the practice of oncology to undergraduates and oncology trainees. As we watched our students moving 'along the learning curve', we perceived a gap in the available learning resources. Students read large and authoritative textbooks of oncology presenting extensive information and data reviews, but still struggle when faced with a clinical scenario and asked: 'What would you do for this patient and why?'

It was our aim to produce a text which would help students cross the gap between theory and practice. We chose a 'case-based' format to impart a sense of reality to the learning process, and hopefully to combine evidence with the wisdom of experience.

Chapter 1 (Basic science of oncology), presents clinically relevant data from molecular biology, statistics and trial analysis, and quality of life research. This chapter includes a guide to oncology information and evidence databases on the Internet. The focus is on what practising clinicians should know, but might have difficulty finding elsewhere in a digestible form.

Chapter 2 (Making management decisions) presents the principles which guide decision making in oncology. Integration of tumour factors, patient factors, and treatment factors into the decision making process is emphasized.

Cancer management requires the skills of a variety of clinicians: surgical oncologists, radiation oncologists, medical oncologists, palliative care physicians, oncology nurses, and others. The integration of these disciplines into the overall management of each major tumour type has been emphasized in subsequent chapters. The reality of oncology practice requires the inclusion of issues in supportive care and symptom control.

The final chapter (Managing the end of life) deals with issues such as 'Breaking bad news', 'Dealing with angry patients', and 'Managing the last 48 hours of life'. Skills in these areas are as vital to the outcome of care for an individual patient and his/her carers as are the surgery and radiation or chemotherapy they receive.

Finally, it is our earnest hope that this book will prove enticing and satisfying to the reader. We could have no greater satisfaction than to think that a trainee will see the cases in this book and think: 'I need to read this!'

Sydney, Australia   P.H., J.C., and P.G.
1999

Acknowledgements

We sincerely thank the many busy clinicians and scientists who have given of their time, experience, and wisdom in contributing to this work.

We especially thank Jennifer Butler and Rosemary Cartmill for their major contributions to the production of this book.

List of contributors

Verity Ann Ahern MBBS, FRACR, Staff Specialist, Department of Radiation Oncology, Westmead Hospital, Westmead NSW 2145, Australia, Ph: +61-2-9845 6499, Fax: +61-2-9891 5814, Email: veritya@bci.org.au

John Boyages MB BS (Hons) (Syd) FRACR PhD, Associate Professor, Executive Director, NSW Breast Cancer Institute, Westmead Hospital, Westmead NSW 2145, Australia, Phone: 61-2 9845 8458, Fax: 61-2 9845 8491, email: johnb@bci.org.au

Steven Boyages MB BS DDU FRACP FAFPHM PhD, Clinical Associate Professor, University of Sydney, Director, Department of Diabetes and Endocrinology, Westmead Hospital, Westmead NSW 2145, Australia, Ph: +61-2-9845 8180, Fax: +61-2-9635 5691, Email: steveb@westgate.wh. usyd.edu.au

Michael Boyer MB BS, PhD, FRACP, Department Head, Department of Medical Oncology, Sydney Cancer Centre, Royal Prince Alfred Hospital, Camperdown NSW 2050, Phone 61-2-9515 5494, Fax 61-2-9519 1546, E-mail mboyer@canc.rpa.cs.nsw.gov.au

Rhonda Brown BSc PhD, Medical Psychology Unit, Department of Psychological Medicine, University of Sydney, Royal North Shore Hospital, Medical Psychology Unit, Building 82, level 10, Royal Prince Alfred Hospital, Camperdown NSW 2050, Australia, Ph: +61-2-951565800, Fax: +61-2-95155697, Email: medpsych@mail.usyd.edu.au

Colin A Bull MBBS, FRCR, FRACR, Director Radiation Oncology, Westmead and Nepean Hospitals, Joint Radiation Oncology Centre (JROC), Westmead NSW 2145, Australia, Ph: +61-2-9845 6489, Fax: +61-2-9891 5814, e-mail: bull@radonc.wsahs.nsw.gov.au

Phyllis Butow BA(Hons) M Clin Psych MPH, PhD, Executive Director, Medical Psychology Unit, Department of Psychological Medicine, University of Sydney and, Research Co-ordinator, Dept of Psychological Medicine, Royal North Shore Hospital, Medical Psychology Unit, Building 82, level 10, Royal Prince Alfred Hospital, Camperdown NSW 2050, Australia, Ph +61-2-9515 7097, Fax: +61-2-9515 5697, email: medpsych @mail.usyd.edu.au

John Cartmill MB BS BSc(med) MM FRACS, Senior Lecturer in Surgery, University of Sydney, Staff Specialist Colorectal Surgeon, Nepean Hospital, PO Box 63, Penrith NSW 2751, Australia, Ph: +61-2-4724 3136, Fax: +61-2-4724 3242

Felix Chan FRACOG, Staff Specialist, Department of Gynaecological Oncology, Westmead Hospital, Westmead NSW 2145, Australia, Ph: 9845 6801, Fax: 9845 7793, Email: Felixc@westmead.wsahs.nsw.gov.au

Richard Chye MBBS (Syd), FRACP, Director, Palliative Care, South Eastern Sydney Area Health Service, Sacred Heart Hospice, 170 Darlinghurst Road, Darlinghurst, Sydney NSW 2010, Australia, Ph: +61-2-9361 9444, Fax : +61-2-9361 9518, email : rchye@stvincents.com.au

John Collins MBBS PhD, FRACP, Physician, Vincent Fairfax Pain Unit, The New Children's Hospital, Westmead NSW 2145, Australia, Ph: +61-2-9845000 Pge 6415, Fax: +61-2-9845 3421, Email: johnc4@nch.edu.au

Neil Cooney MB BS, FRACP, Staff Specialist, Palliative Care Institute, St Vincent's Hospital, 170 Darlinghurst Road, Darlinghurst NSW 2010, Australia, Ph: +61-2-9361 9444, Fax: +61-2-9361 9518, Ncooney@stvincents.com.au

Michael Cox MB BS, MS FRACS, Staff Specialist Surgeon, Nepean Hospital, PO Box 63, Penrith, 2751, Australia, Ph: +61-2-4724 2607, Fax: +61-2-4724 3432

Peter Cox FANZCA, Visiting Anaesthetist, Pain Management Consultant, Westmead Hospital, Westmead, NSW, 2145, Australia, Ph: +61-2-9845 6447, Fax: +61-2-9810 6762, Email: pwaj@ZIP.com.au

Patrick Cregan FRACS, Breast and Endocrine and Endoscopic Surgery, Nepean Hospital, PO Box 63, Penrith NSW 2751, Australia, Ph: +61-2-4721 4489, Fax: +61-2-47 322698, Email: Patrick_Cregan@onaustralia.com.au

David Currow B Med MPH FRACP, Lecturer in Medicine, University of Sydney, Senior Staff Specialist, Palliative Medicine and Interim Director, Nepean Cancer Care Centre, The Nepean Hospital, PO Box 63, Penrith NSW 2751, Australia, Ph: +61-2-4724 2038, Fax: +61-2-4724 2137, Email: currowd@wahs.health.nsw.gov.au

Anna deFazio BSc. PhD, Senior Scientist, Department of Gynaecological Oncology, Westmead Hospital, Westmead NSW 2145, Australia, Phone: 61-2-9845 7376, Fax: 61-2-9845 7793, Email: annadf@westmed.wh.usyd.edu.au

Michael Frommer MB BS DOBst RCOG MPH FAFOM FAFPHM, Deputy Director, Australian Centre for Effective Healthcare, Associate Professor, Department of Public Health and Community Medicine, University of Sydney, Rm 224/Bldg A27, Sydney NSW 2006, Australia, Tel 61-2-9351-4378, Fax 61-2-9351-5204

Paul Glare MB BS FRACP, Head, Department of Palliative Care, Sydney Cancer Centre, Royal Prince Alfred Hospital, Missenden Road, Camperdown NSW 2050, Australia, Ph: +61-2-9515 3608, Fax: +61-2-9515 3609, Email: paul@pal.rpa.cs.nsw.gov.au

David J Gorman MB BS BSc(Med) FRACP, Calvary Hospital, PO Box 261, Kogarah NSW 2217, Australia, Phone: +61-2-295878333, Fax: +61-2-95881635, Email: DavidG@sesahs.nsw.gov.au

Howard Gurney MB BS, FRACP, Staff Specialist, Department of Medical Oncology and Palliative Care, Westmead Hospital, Westmead NSW 2145, Australia, Ph: +61-2-9845 6954, Fax: +61-2-9845 6391, Email: howardG@westmed.wh.usyd.edu.au

Jane Hall BA (Econ) PhD, Associate Professor, Director, CHERE, Level 6, Bldg F, 88 Mallett St, Camperdown NSW 2050, Australia, Ph: +61-2-9351 0900, Fax: +61-2-9351 0930, Email: janeh@chere.usyd.edu.au

Richard Halliwell MB BS, FANZCA, Clinical Lecturer, Department of Anaesthesia, University of Sydney, Westmead Hospital, Westmead, NSW, 2145, Australia, Ph: +61-2-9845 6447, Fax: +61-2-9633 3764, Email: richardh@westgate.wh.usyd.edu.au

Paul R Harnett MB BS FRACP PhD, Clinical Associate Professor, University of Sydney, Director Department of Medical Oncology and Palliative Care, Westmead Hospital, Westmead NSW 2145, Australia, Ph: +61-2-9845 6954, Fax: +61-2-9845 6391, Email: harnettpr@hemonc.wh.su.edu.au

Michael Henderson MB BS, BmedSc, MD, FRACS, University of Melbourne Department of Surgery, St Vincent's Hospital, Department of Surgical Oncology, St Vincent's Hospital and Peter MacCallum Cancer Institute, 41 Victoria Parade, Fitzroy, 3065, Australia, Ph: +6-13-9288 2545, Fax: +6-13-9288 2571, Email: henderson@surgerysvh.unimelb.edu.au

Mark S. Hertzberg MB BS PhD FRACP FRCPA, Senior Staff Specialist Department of Haematology, Westmead Hospital, Westmead NSW, 2145, Australia, Ph: +61-2-9845 6274, Fax: +61-2-9689 2331, Email: markh@westmed.wh.usyd.edu.au

Peter Hewitt MB BS FRACS, Head of Department of Colorectal Surgery, Division of Surgery, North Western Adelaide Health Service, The Queen Elizabeth Hospital, 28 Woodville Road, Woodville South, 5011, Australia, Ph: +61-8-8222 6248, Fax: +61-8-8222 6028, Email: phewett@tqehsmtp.tqeh.sa.gov.au

T. Michael D. Hughes MB BS FRACS, Fellow in Surgical Oncology, Melanoma and Sarcoma Unit, Royal Marsden Hospital, Fulham Rd, London SW3 6JJ UK, Email: tmdhughes@hotmail.com

Richard F. Kefford MB BS PhD FRACP, Professor of Medicine and Director, Westmead Institute for Cancer Research, University of Sydney at Westmead Hospital, Westmead NSW 2145, Australia, Phone: +61-2-9845-6033, Fax: +61-2-9687-2331, Email: kefford@westgate.wh.usyd.edu.au

Judy Kirk MB BS FRACP, Senior Staff Specialist in Cancer Genetics, Familial Cancer Service, Department of Medicine, University of Sydney, Westmead Hospital, Westmead NSW 2145, Ph: +61-2-98455079, Fax: +61-2-9687 2331, Email: judyk@westgate.wh.usyd.edu.au

Howard M H Lau MBBS (Syd Uni) FRACS (Urol), Consultant Urologist and Transplant Surgeon, Department of Surgery, Westmead Hospital, Westmead NSW 2145, Australia, Ph: +61-2- 9845 6821, Email: hlau@bigpond.com

Peter B Loder FRACS, Colorectal Surgeon, Visiting Medical Officer, Department of Surgery, Westmead Hospital, Suite 1-10, 10 Edgeworth David Ave, Hornsby NSW 2077, Australia, Ph: +61-2-9477 7948, Fax: +61-2-9477 7183, Email: Peter.Loder@hcn.net.au

Craig MacLeod FRACR (radiation oncology), Staff Specialist, Department of Radiation Oncology, Sydney Cancer Centre, Royal Prince Alfred Hospital, Missenden Rd, Camperdown NSW 2050, Australia, Phone +61-2-9515-8059, Fax +61-2-9515-8115, Email: cmacleod@radonc.rpa.cs.nsw.gov.au

Graham J Mann MBBS PhD FRACP, Senior Lecturer in Medicine, University of Sydney, Westmead Institute of Cancer Research, Westmead Hospital, Westmead NSW 2145, Australia, Ph: 61-2-9845-6494, Fax: 61-2-9845-8319, Email: gmann@mail.usyd.edu.au

Glenn M Marshall MB BS, FRACP, MD, Head, Division Of Haematology, and Oncology, Associate Professor in Paediatrics, Level 1 Sydney Children's Hospital, High St, Randwick 2031, Australia, Ph: +61-2-9382 1721, Fax: +61-2-9382 1789, Email: G.Marshall@unsw.edu.au

Christopher Martin MB BS MSc FRACS, Professor of Surgery, University of Sydney, Head of Surgery, Nepean Hospital, PO Box 63, Penrith NSW 2751, Australia, Ph: +61-2-47 242608, Fax: +61-2-47 243432

Jane Mathews BSc (Hons) PhD A.Stat, Statistical Centre, Peter McCallum Cancer Institute, St Andrews Place, East Melbourne, VIC 3002, Australia, Ph: +61-3-9656 1268, Email: janem@petermac.unimelb.edu.au

Geoffrey McCowage FRACP, Staff Specialist, Department of Oncology, The New Children's Hospital, PO Box 3515, Parramatta NSW 2124, Australia, Ph: (61)-2-9845-2122, Fax: (61)-2-9845-2171, Email: GeoffM@nch.edu.au

Alan P Meagher FRACS, Colorectal Surgeon, Department of Surgery, St Vincent's Hospital, Victoria St, Darlinghurst NSW 2010, Australia, Ph: +61-2-93326681, Fax +61-2-9332 6679

Gary Morgan FRACDS FRACS, General Surgeon, Head & Neck Surgery, Department of Surgery, Westmead Hospital, Westmead NSW 2145, Australia, Ph: +61-2-9845 6886, Fax: +61-2-9893 7440, Email: c_gmorgan@bigpond.com.au

Michael Morgan MD (Syd) FRACS, Professor of Neurosurgery, Royal North Shore Hospital, Department of Neurosurgery, Level 7, Royal North Shore Hospital, St Leonards NSW 2065, Australia, Ph: +61-2-9926 8756, Fax: +61-2-9437 5172, Email: morgan@med.usyd.edu.au

Stephen P. Mulligan, MB BS (Hons), Ph.D., FRACP, FRCPA, Department of Haematology, Concord Hospital NSW 2139, Australia, Ph: +61-2-9767-6651, Fax: +61-2-9676-7650, Email: mulligan@mpx.com.au

George Rubin MB BS, FRACP, FAFPHM, FACPM, FACE, Director, Effective Healthcare Australia (EHA), Professor of Public Health and Community Medicine, University of Sydney at Westmead, Rm 224/Bldg A27 NSW 2006, Sydney NSW 2006, Australia, Ph: +61-2-9351-4378, Fax +61-2-9351-5204, Email: grubin@dph1.health.usyd.edu.au

Christopher Ryan MBBS (Hons), FRANZCP, Staff Specialist in Consultation-Liaison Psychiatry, Westmead Hospital, University of Sydney, Westmead NSW 2145, Australia, Ph: +61-2-9845 6688, Fax: +61-2-9635 7734, Email: cryan@mail.usyd.edu.au

Lali H. S. Sekhon MB BS (Hons), PhD, FRACS, Neurosurgery Fellow, Department of Neurological Surgery, Mayo Clinic, Rochester, Minnesota, USA, Ph: +1-507-2555123, Fax: +1-507-2552249, Email: lali@lali.com.au

Jennifer Shannon FRACP, Department of Medical Oncology, Westmead Hospital, Westmead NSW 2145, Australia, Ph: +61-2-9845 6954, Fax: +61-2-9845-8319, Email: jennys@hemonc.wh.su.edu.au

Howard Smith MB BS BSc(Med) FRACP PhD(ANU), Director Westmead Fertility Centre, Senior Staff Specialist, Dept. Clinical Endocrinology, Westmead Hospital, Westmead NSW 2145, Australia, Ph: +61-2-9845 6796, Fax: +61-2-9635 5691, Email: howards@westmed. wh.usyd.edu.au

Michael Solomon MB BCH BAO (Hons) LRCSE LRCPI MSc FRACS, Clinical Associate Professor, Department of Surgery, University of Sydney, Colorectal Unit, Royal Prince Alfred Hospital, Missenden Rd, Camperdown NSW 2050, Australia, Ph: +61-2-9519 7576, Fax: +61-2-9519 1806

Odette Spruyt MB ChB Dip Obs FRACP, Director, Pain and Palliative Care Service, Peter McCallum Cancer Institute, St Andrews Place, East Melbourne, Vic 3002, Australia, Ph: +61-3-9656 1265, Fax: +61-3-9656 1408, Email: odettespruyt@petermac.unimelb.edu.au

Bruce Stafford MB BS FRACP Grad Cert in Health (Palliative Care), Medical Officer, Palliative Care Department, Mater Hospital, South Brisbane, Queensland, 4101, Ph: +61-7-3840 8873, Fax: +61-7-3840 8277

Ken Tiver MB BS (Syd) FRACR, Deputy Director, Joint Radiation Oncology Centre, Cancer Care Centre, Nepean Hospital, PO Box 63, Penrith, NSW, 2751, Australia, Ph: +61-2-4724 2363, Fax: +61-2-4724 3570

Sandra Turner MB BS (Hons) (Syd), FRACR, Staff Specialist, Dept. Radiation Oncology, Westmead Hospital, Westmead NSW 2145, Australia, Ph: +61-2-9845 6499, Fax: +61-2- 98195814, Email: turner@radonc.wsahs.nsw.gov.au

Owen A Ung FRACS, Breast & Endocrine Surgeon, Clinical Services Director, NSW Breast Cancer Institute, Westmead Hospital, Westmead NSW 2145, Australia, Ph: +61-2-9845 8464, Fax: +61-2-9845 7246, Email: owenu@bci.org.au

Gerard V. Wain FRACOG CGO, Director of Gynaecological Oncology Department, Westmead Hospital, Westmead, NSW 2145, Australia, Ph: +61-2-9845 6801, Fax: +61-2-9845 8311, Email: gerardw@ westmead.wsahs.nsw.gov.au

Nicholas Wilcken MB BS, FRACP, PhD, Staff Specialist, Department of Medical Oncology and Palliative Care, Westmead Hospital, Westmead NSW 2145, Australia, Ph +61-2-9845 6954, Fax: +61-2-9845 6391, Email: nicholasw@westmed.wh.usyd.edu.au

Jennifer Wiltshire MBBcH, BAO, CIPM, Area Director Palliative Care South Western Sydney Area Health Service, Clinical Associate Lecturer,

University of NSW, Braeside Hospital, Locked Bag 82, Wetherill Park NSW 2164, Australia, Ph: +61-02-9616 8649, Fax +61-2-9616 8657, Email: j.wiltshire@unsw.edu.au

Noel Young FRACR, Staff Specialist, Department of Radiology, Westmead Hospital, Westmead NSW 2145, Australia, Ph: +61-2-9845 6522, Fax: +61-2-9687 2109

Basic science of oncology

1.1 What are oncogenes and what role do they play in human cancer?

Oncogenes are best understood in an historical context. In one of the classic, early experiments in molecular biology (in the early 1970s), investigators designed a model system to try to isolate mutated genes which caused cancer (i.e. the 'oncogenes'). At that time, it was possible to force small pieces of DNA into mammalian cells (often mouse fibroblasts) growing in tissue culture dishes (the process of 'transfection'). The recipient mammalian cells then expressed the transfected gene, and the resultant effects upon the cultured cells could be studied. When DNA from normal tissue was transfected into mouse fibroblasts (Fig. 1.1A), recipient cells maintained their normal growth characteristics in culture (i.e. benign appearing cytology, limited survival in culture, strict requirements for growth factors in the culture medium, inhibition of mitosis by contact with a neighbouring cell, and an absolute requirement for anchorage to the tissue culture dish for cell division—in short, the features we associate with normal tissues). However, if DNA derived from tumour cell lines was transfected (Fig. 1.1B), colonies of recipient cells with altered cell properties (abnormal cytology, loss of cell–cell contact inhibition, decreased requirement for growth factors in the culture medium, ability to grow indefinitely in culture, anchorage-independent cell division) were detected. The transfected gene had conferred on the recipient cells the features of the malignant phenotype—hence the term oncogene. Further detailed study of the genes which conferred this malignant phenotype revealed that these 'oncogenes' were in fact mutated forms of normal genes found in all cells. However, since the term oncogene had already been conferred on the mutated genes, the normal genes were named, in retrospect, **proto-oncogenes**.

Over 100 normal proto-oncogenes have now been described. Broadly they can be divided into three classes:

1. Proto-oncogenes which code for proteins involved in the transfer of signals from the cell membrane to the nucleus, e.g. the *ras* family (first discovered in viruses that cause *rat sarcomas*); the *trk* (*tropomyosin receptor kinase*) oncogene which encodes the nerve growth factor receptor; *MET* oncogene (identified as an activating oncogene in tumours

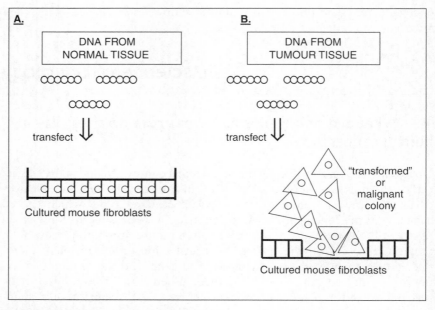

Fig. 1.1 An assay to isolate oncogenes.

caused by the chemical MNNG) which encodes hepatocyte growth factor receptor; *fms* (discovered in viruses that cause *f*eline *s*arcomas) which encodes the colony stimulating factor (CSF-1) receptor.

2. Proto-oncogenes which code for extracellular growth factors, e.g. the *sis* proto-oncogene (discovered in viruses that caused sarcomas in monkeys —*si*mian *s*arcoma) which codes for platelet derived growth factor (PDGF), associated with gliomas.

3. Proto-oncogenes which encode transcription factors that bind to specific sites on DNA, thus activating expression of a particular set of genes, e.g. the *myc* group (discovered in viruses that cause *my*elo*cy*toma in chickens).

It is easy to see how illegitimate activation of such proteins might lead to the malignant phenotype. For example a mutation in a growth factor receptor gene may result in a receptor which is activated even in the absence of its normal ligand, thus providing a perpetual growth stimulus to the cell. A similar effect results from mutations in ras proteins, which are one of the commonest mutations in cancers. Faulty regulation of oncogenes leading to increased production of growth factors (e.g. platelet-derived growth factor—PDGF, transforming growth factor alpha—TGF-α, colony-stimulating factors—CSFs), and/or their cognate receptors, are common in human tumours. There is, therefore, no single normal cellular 'proto-oncogene' function. Rather, the definition embraces any gene which, when mutated, confers a selectable growth or survival advantage on cells in a dominant fashion; that is overriding the activity of any remaining normal copy of that gene.

Mutated proto-oncogenes have been detected in a wide variety of human tumours, and are selected for during the carcinogenic process. However, a single mutated oncogene is rarely sufficient to confer the full malignant phenotype, and mutations in other genes such as tumour suppressor genes and DNA repair genes act in concert with oncogenes in tumorigenesis.

Germline mutations of oncogenes are a very rare cause of *inherited* cancer susceptibility, only two examples being known to date. Mutations in the *RET* proto-oncogene are responsible for several cancer syndromes, including MEN IIA and IIB (multiple endocrine neoplasia syndrome), and familial medullary carcinoma of the thyroid, as well as Hirchsprung's disease. Some rare familial melanoma kindreds carry a mutated form of the cell cycle regulating enzyme Cdk4 (cyclin dependent kinase), which is abnormally sensitive to its own regulator, the p16Cdk4 inhibitor.

Some abnormal proto-oncogenes also have direct clinical significance. For example amplification (i.e. too many copies) of the *N-MYC* oncogene is a highly significant indicator of poor prognosis in childhood neuro-blastoma. Moreover, since mutated proto-oncogenes are tumour specific, experimental therapies directed at abnormal oncogenes and/or their products appear promising.

Of particular interest is recent evidence that antibodies to the erbB-2 oncogene product (overexpressed in about 20 per cent of breast cancers) induce protracted tumour responses in patients with metastatic breast cancer with little toxicity, and the combinations of such antibodies with cytotoxic chemotherapy increased response rates. Moreover, vaccination with synthetic peptides constructed to resemble the erbB-2 protein can induce an immune response in breast cancer patients, stimulating hopes for effective immunotherapy for breast cancer, or even other tumours.

1.2 What are tumour suppressor genes and what role do they play in human cancer?

Cancer is best regarded as a cellular phenotype resulting from critical losses of various functions controlling cellular lifespan, proliferative potential, genomic integrity, and normal tissue architecture.

Historically speaking, tumour suppressor genes were identified on the basis that they were inactivated by mutation in tumours and that they could suppress the malignant phenotype if artificially reintroduced into tumour cell lines in culture. Sequential 'hits' to both copies of the gene (since human cells carry two copies of every gene, except on the sex chromosomes) occur during tumour development, resulting in a strong selective growth advantage for cells with complete loss of these functions. Tumour suppressor genes do not encode proteins with an 'antitumorigenesis' function, since 'antitumorigenesis' is not a physiological function in the usual sense.

Over 30 tumour suppressor genes have been identified to date. Mutations in the suppressor gene *p53* (located on chromosome 17) are the commonest mutations found in human cancer. The normal *p53* gene product plays a pivotal role in a variety of cellular processes, including the regulation of the mitotic cycle, detection and repair of DNA damage, and regulation of apoptosis. Given the importance of *p53* in cellular homeostasis, it is straightforward to visualize how impaired function of *p53* may contribute to the malignant phenotype.

Abnormalities in tumour suppressor genes can also be inherited. In the case of the rare familial cancer syndromes, abnormalities of specific suppressor genes are *inherited*, so that every cell in the body in the affected offspring is deficient in the function of a specific suppressor gene (e.g. the *BRCA1* gene in familial breast cancer kindreds, the *RB* or retinoblastoma gene in familial retinoblastoma kindreds). These children are at high risk of developing specific cancers. However, since the mutation is in fact carried by every cell in the body, such individuals are predisposed to bilateral tumours that typically occur at a relatively young age.

Table 1.1 Suppressor genes and associated tumours

Suppressor gene	Cellular function	Associated tumours	Chromosomal location
p53	multiple roles in cell cycle control, regulation of apoptosis, DNA damage repair	Li–Fraumeni syndrome—astrocytomas, breast, colon, lung osteosarcoma	17q12–13.3
BRCA1	? DNA repair	breast	17q21
BRCA2	? DNA repair	breast, ovarian, prostate	
NF1 (Neurofibromatosis Type 1)	intracellular signalling	neurofibromas, CNS tumours	17q11.2
WT1	encodes a DNA-binding protein which regulates other genes	Wilms tumour	11p13
APC (adenomatous polyposis coli)	unknown	colorectal, other GIT and CNS tumours	5q21–22
Ptc *NBCCs* (nevoid basal cell carcinoma or Gorlins syndrome)	unknown	basal cell carcinomas, medulloblastomas, and ovarian fibromas	9q23
CDKN2A	cell cycle control	melanoma, pancreatic cancer (leukaemia, lung cancer if somatic as well)	9p21

Studies of familial cancers have generally pointed to tumour suppressor genes with a strong, sometimes exclusive, relationship to cancers of a specific tissue type (see Table 1.1). This has led to the proposal that their inactivation (e.g. of the *PTC* gene in the development of basal cell carcinoma, or the *APC* or *a*denomatous *p*olyposis *c*oli gene in colonic adenomas) is critically important for subsequent tumorigenesis, hence their designation as 'gatekeeper genes'. In contrast, genes concerned with genome integrity (e.g. *p53*, the DNA-mismatch repair genes, etc.) fulfil 'caretaker' roles which mitigate against carcinogenesis across a broader range of tumour types. These actions may not be mutually exclusive.

Understanding the function of tumour suppressor genes opens up the prospect of tumour-specific genetic therapy. Important first steps have been taken towards this goal. It has been established that supplementation of tumour cells with additional suppressor gene products (e.g. by transfection of *BRCA1* or *p53* into tumour cells lacking these genes/proteins) effectively switches off the malignant phenotype. However, many technical problems remain to be solved before such approaches become effective therapy (specific delivery of the therapeutic gene to the tumour cells, controlled and sustained expression of the gene, etc.). Initial clinical trials of such gene therapies are underway.

1.3 What is the relevance of DNA damage and repair to carcinogenesis and cancer therapy?

Severe damage to DNA may trigger a cell to undergo apoptosis as an adaptive response to protect the whole organism. Lesser degrees of DNA damage may be consistent with cell survival but, if not repaired before cell division, will result in the establishment of a mutant clone of cells which may acquire further mutations and ultimately become malignant.

An important component of the normal response to DNA damage is a pause in progression through the cell cycle to allow time to repair accumulated DNA damage. These pauses or 'checkpoint controls' occur at the G_1/S and G_2/M boundaries, and are regulated by a number of genes, including the tumour suppressor genes *p53* and *ATM*. DNA damage induces *p53* accumulation, which in turn sets in motion a cascade of gene expression, including a protein known as *p21* (also known as WAF1 or CIP1) which inhibits cyclins, thus retarding progress through the G_1/S checkpoint. Another *p53*-induced gene, *GADD45* appears to be involved in the specific repair of DNA damage, thus emphasizing the pivotal role *p53* plays in cell cycle control, DNA repair, and apoptosis.

A number of rare inherited disorders characterized by defective repair of DNA damage are associated with cancer predisposition. Ataxia telangiectasia (AT) is a rare, inherited disorder characterized by predisposition to lymphoid neoplasms and abnormal sensitivity to ionizing radiation. Cell lines from normal tissues from people with AT show defects in their ability to pause at G1/S, S, and G2/M checkpoints. Moreover, the cloned AT gene shows structural similarities to yeast checkpoint control genes. Xeroderma pigmentosum is a rare, recessive disorder caused by an inability to repair DNA damaged by ultraviolet irradiation, and is associated with an extraordinarily high incidence of cutaneous malignancy. Fanconi's anaemia (characterized by sensitivity to DNA cross-linking agents) and Bloom's syndrome (in which a defect in DNA helicase activity leads to increased frequency of spontaneous chromosome breakage) are other examples.

Perhaps numerically more important are defects in the cellular processes which repair sequence mismatches in DNA. Normally, base pairing in DNA is tightly regulated, such that A pairs with T only, and C pairs with G only. Should any errors occur, the resultant base mismatches are rapidly repaired by a series of enzymes known as the DNA mismatch repair system. Individuals with defects in mismatch repair are prone to hereditary non-polyposis colon cancer (HNPCC). This syndrome, which accounts for approximately 1 to 6 per cent of colon cancer, exists in two autosomal dominant forms (Lynch I—proximal colon tumours, and Lynch II—multiple colonic, breast, and genitourinary adenocarcinomas). Mutations in mismatch repair genes *hMSH2*, *hMLH1*, *hPMS1*, and *hPMS2* have been described in HNPCC kindreds and also in sporadic cases of colon cancer. Such defects in mismatch repair lead to what is known as 'microsatellite instability' (detectable on gel electrophoresis of PCR amplified DNA), in which areas of the genome containing simple repetitive sequences (e.g. GC.GC.GC.GC) become longer or shorter than normal. If such altered length sequences happen to occur within critical genes, abnormal gene expression may result, with ensuing colon carcinogenesis.

Since most cytotoxic drugs and therapeutic ionizing radiation kill cells by damaging DNA, it is not surprising that DNA repair processes play a role in determining tumour response to therapy. At least in cultured tumour cell lines, increased activity of some repair pathways confers relative resistance to cytotoxics or irradiation. Paradoxically, impaired repair of DNA-mismatches is associated with relative resistance to some drugs, notably cisplatin. Elucidation of such processes is a burgeoning field in cancer research.

1.4 What happens to tumour cells which are responding to therapy?

Cells may die by one of two processes, necrosis or apoptosis. In necrotic cell death (typified by hypoxic cells as seen in myocardial infarction) cells undergo reduced energy (i.e. ATP) levels, loss of functional integrity of the cell membrane, and subsequent cellular swelling. Necrotic cell death effects large groups of cells within a tissue, is associated with a marked inflammatory host response, and is usually painful.

By contrast, tumours responding to therapy are generally not painful or inflamed, and seem to melt away in an asymptomatic fashion. Tumours responding to chemotherapy, irradiation, or hormonal therapy undergo an active self-destruction process known as apoptosis. The process of apoptosis also underlies regression of lactating breasts after weaning, and even the resorption of a tadpole's tail as it matures. During apoptosis, individual cells activate an energy-requiring programme of self-lysis performed by specific endonucleases and proteases. Apoptosis is not associated with an inflammatory response. A hallmark of apoptosis is digestion of DNA into fragments that are multiples of 160 base pairs in size, seen as DNA ladders by gel electrophoresis.

Apoptosis can be triggered by DNA damage (e.g. by cytotoxics or irradiation), by growth factor withdrawal (e.g. ablation of testosterone in prostatic carcinoma), by corticosteroids (e.g. lymphoma), or by heat shock. The mechanisms for sensing such triggers are complex and involve several proteins. High levels of $p53$ protein (which accumulate in late G1 after DNA damage) can trigger apoptosis. Tumour cells lacking in $p53$ have a higher threshold for undergoing apoptosis (i.e. are relatively resistant) after DNA damage by chemotherapy or irradiation. However, $p53$ independent pathways also exist.

A family of genes exists whose function is to regulate the induction of apoptosis. The protein bax triggers apoptosis, whereas the related protein Bcl-2 blocks this pathway. The balance between these two proteins is a critical determinant of the outcome of DNA damage and therefore impacts upon both tumorigenesis and cancer treatment. For example cells with abnormally high levels of Bcl-2 may be more likely to metastasize and have a poor prognosis. High expression of bax in ovarian cancer is associated with prolonged response to paclitaxel-containing chemotherapy. Identification of the factors which affect apoptosis has obvious relevance to cancer therapy, and investigation into agents which might modulate this pathway (e.g. caspase inhibitors) is an area of intense research.

1.5 Retrospective comparisons of treatments

Three years ago an Oncology Centre introduced a new treatment (treatment B) for patients with a particular type of cancer. In the preceding 5 years the Centre had used treatment A for these patients. In order to assess the benefits of the new treatment, the Centre wishes to compare the results of all patients treated with treatment A with those of patients treated with treatment B.

What are the potential sources of bias? Can these be minimized or avoided?
The first potential source of bias is **selection bias**. The patients selected to receive treatment B may not have the same prognosis as the patients selected to receive treatment A. This is most likely to be a problem when treatment B is associated with more toxicity than treatment A and thus may be restricted to younger/fitter patients. This could make the results for treatment B look better than the results for treatment A just because patients with a better prognosis have been treated with B. A possible solution is to compare the results of all patients with the particular cancer who presented during the 3-year period when treatment B was available with the results for all patients with that cancer who presented during the preceding 5-year period. Thus we would essentially test whether the availability of treatment B in the centre has improved the prognosis of the relevant patients.

In order to ascribe any changes in results in the two periods to the availability of treatment B, it would have to be assumed that there were no other relevant changes in the two time periods. Better supportive care could improve the results for the more recent patients leading to a **temporal bias**. More refined diagnostic tools could lead to **assessment bias** if a 'soft' endpoint based on disease response or progression were chosen. An increased probability of detecting residual disease could decrease the response rate and decrease the time to failure or progression. This could be avoided by using overall survival as the primary endpoint.

Assessment bias could also be an issue if results were compared only for patients with a particular stage. More refined diagnostic tools could lead to patients being 'up-staged', that is assigned a higher stage category than would have been assigned without the more refined tools. This can lead to an apparent improvement in results in a stage by stage comparison simply due to the influx of better prognosis patients in the higher stages and the efflux of the worse prognosis patients from the lower stages (the so-called 'Will Rogers' phenomenon after the ascribed quotation: 'When the Okies left Oklahoma and moved to California they raised the average intelligence level in both States'). Again this can be avoided by comparing the results for all patients during the two periods, not just patients with selected stages.

Changes in referral patterns during the time periods under study could also lead to a bias. If treatment B were a highly promising and well-publicized treatment being tested in a clinical trial at the Oncology Centre, referrals to the Centre might increase during the period of availability of B. The extra patients being referred might have a different prognosis than the patients who are usually referred. Rates of referral and patient characteristics could be compared for the two time periods and methods of analysis which adjust for differences in baseline characteristics could be used in the comparison of results, but for these to be valid it would be essential to ensure that there were no assessment biases leading to differences in measuring the characteristics.

Although the appropriate steps can be taken to make the comparison of the two treatments as valid as possible in the given circumstances, only a properly conducted, randomized trial comparing treatment A and treatment B can eliminate all sources of bias.

1.6 Comparisons of responders and non-responders

A new chemotherapy regimen has been tested on a series of patients. To demonstrate the efficacy of the regimen, the survival of patients who respond to the new regimen are compared with the survival of patients who have failed to respond.

Is it valid to compare the survival of responders and non-responders?
It is not valid to compare the survival of responders and non-responders directly, that is by drawing a survival curve for the responders and a survival curve for the non-responders and comparing these two curves. In order to be assessed and classified as a responder, a patient has to have survived a certain minimum amount of time. The time will depend on the definition of response and the timing of the response assessment. For example if the response is to be assessed by a CT scan 4 weeks after completion of the third course of treatment and treatments are given every 4 weeks, then in order to be a responder a patient will need to survive at least 12 weeks from the beginning of treatment. If the response criteria specify that the response must be maintained for at least 4 weeks, then a responder will have a minimum survival of 16 weeks, just by definition. All patients who die within the first 16 weeks will be classified as non-responders, although some might have become responders if they had survived long enough. Even if the non-responders that survive 16 weeks have exactly the same subsequent survival as the responders, the overall survival following commencement of treatment for the group of non-responders will be less than that of the group of responders because of the early deaths in the group of non-responders.

One valid way to compare responders with non-responders is to perform a 'landmark' analysis, in which only patients who have survived a particular time are compared. In the example above only the group of patients who survived 16 weeks could be studied. The survival of those who were classified as responders by that time could then be compared with the survival of those who were classified as non-responders at that time. This group might include some patients who subsequently become responders. In order to include the patients whose assessments might have been delayed, for example through delays in receiving treatment, a time-point later than 16 weeks might be chosen, say 18 or 20 weeks, or even the latest observed time to achieve response in the group of patients under study. However, if the time-point is too far away from the commencement of treatment, too much data may be made uninformative and the comparison may lack statistical power.

An alternative and more powerful statistical method of comparing the survival of responders and non-responders is to use a Cox proportional hazards regression model with time dependent covariates. In this model a patient is classified as a non-responder until the time that he or she becomes a responder. Thus the patient belongs to the 'risk set' of the non-responders until he or she achieves a response and then transfers to the 'risk set' of the responders. For this method to be valid the Cox proportional hazards model would need to provide an adequate description of the data.

If the responders survive longer than the non-responders, can their improved prognosis be attributed to their treatment?

If it is validly shown that the responding patients have a better survival than the non-responding patients do, it does not necessarily follow that their better survival is attributable to their response to the treatment. It is possible that patients who respond to treatment have a better prognosis than patients who do not respond. Similarly the longer survival of the responding patients does not imply that the treatment in itself is effective.

1.7 What is the difference between quality of life and 'QALY's?

Maintaining quality of life is an important aspect of the management of individual cancer patients. Health-related quality of life is increasingly a focus of clinical trials and here specific measures of quality of life are required as endpoints. These measures have three essential features:

- they are about health;
- they are subjective, the patient's own perception of their health;
- they are multidimensional encompassing physical, emotional, and social aspects.

Each dimension is measured separately and, in general, these are not combined to give a single score. An individual's rating on a dimension is expressed as a numeric score, often on an arbitrary scale of 1 to 100.

QALY stands for 'quality *a*djusted *l*ife *y*ear'. The idea was developed as an outcome measure for economic evaluation. So, to understand the QALY, one must first know something about economic evaluation. Economic evaluation is the comparison of two alternatives in terms of their costs and benefits. Suppose a new cancer treatment is developed. Is it better or worse than the conventional treatment? Economic evaluation assesses the benefits, in general the improvement in survival, with the costs of the new treatment over the old. The most widely used form of economic evaluation is cost effectiveness analysis. Benefits are measured as life years gained; costs are measured in money; and the two treatments can be compared in terms of the cost per life year gained. For example Smith *et al.*, showed that adjuvant chemotherapy for Dukes' C colonic carcinoma cost an additional $7000 (Australian $) per patient for a gain of 2.4 life years, that is approximately $2900 per life year gained. The problem with cost effectiveness analysis is that every life year is treated as equivalent to every other. There are many instances where differences in quality of life are the important outcome to be assessed; or where the comparison of two treatments involves a trade-off between survival and quality of life. In the study by Smith *et al.*, surgical treatment is followed by weekly chemotherapy treatment for 50 weeks. It seems self evident that a year spent having weekly chemotherapy is not the same quality as a year spent feeling fully recovered. A more refined outcome measure would trade off the increase in survival with the decrease in quality of life in a single score.

For many new cancer treatments the appropriate form of economic evaluation is where the measure of benefits combines both quantity and quality of life and this is called 'cost–utility analysis'. The most frequently used measure (but not the only one) is the QALY. QALYs differ from the more familiar measures of quality of life in that the multiple dimensions must be reduced to a single score and the numeric scale that is used must have particular properties. This does not mean that fewer dimensions should be covered, since anything that makes a difference to how patients value their health-related quality of life is relevant. A particular state of quality of life, usually called a health state, can be described in terms of each of the dimensions of quality of life. For each health state, a single numeric score is derived; this is the quality weight given to that state (sometimes called a 'utility'). The numeric score must have special properties, which means it has to be derived using valid methods. First, a year in full health scores 1, and death scores 0. These are the anchor points of the scale. This is so that survival can be adjusted by the quality of life weight. Second, the scale must have interval properties, that is the difference between 0.5 and 0.7 must be equivalent to any difference of 0.2 between any other points on the scale. This is so that the arithmetic manipulation of life years and weights is valid.

There are a number of different methods used to derive QALY weights. These are discussed in several texts. In principle, the number of QALYs can then be estimated by taking the number of life years in each health state, and multiplying that by the QALY weight (although there are further refinements, again, see any text). The difference between considering only life years and quality adjusted life years is illustrated in Fig. 1.2. The number of life years gained is shown on the x axis; therefore the difference in

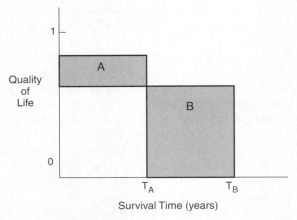

Fig. 1.2 Calculating quality adjusted life years.

survival between two treatments can be measured along that axis, $T_b - T_a$. QALYs are estimated by adjusting each life year by its quality weight and can be calculated as the area under the curve; the difference in QALYs is the difference between the areas under the curve, B–A.

Does adjusting for quality of life make a difference?
Many clinicians have argued that survival is the only important thing to patients; or that when compared to survival, quality of life differences will not have a meaningful effect. In the paper by Smith *et al.*, the quality of life weights used were between 0.8 and 1. Even this relatively small difference has an effect on the results. In terms of QALYs gained, adjuvant chemo-therapy adds 0.4 QALYs (vs. 2.4 life-years) and the cost per QALY is $17,500 (vs. $2900 per life year gained).

There have been various debates about the validity of the methods used to derive QALYs. For example as a patient spends longer in a particular health state, he/she adjusts to it so that his/her quality of life improves even though the health state has not changed. An alternative approach which has been developed is the 'healthy year equivalent', or HYE. There is also debate about the equity implications of QALYs. Some argue that QALYS are egalitarian because a QALY is a QALY no matter whose it is. Others argue that QALYs should be weighted to reflect health system goals in regard to equity. Another variation on the QALY is the 'disability adjusted life year' or DALY which does include some equity weighting. This has been developed in the WHO Global Burden of Disease Project.

There has also been much criticism that QALYs are too narrowly focused. By counting only health outcomes, QALYs are excluding potentially im-portant benefits such as the value of information or the value to patients of being able to take part in treatment decisions. These critics have suggested that a broader metric for measuring benefits is required, and they are exploring the use of cost–benefit analysis where benefits are measured in money. New developments in the health economics literature are likely therefore to move beyond QALYs.

1.8 Accessing electronic information to inform effective clinical practice

Good access to research-based evidence is essential to stay well informed and improve the effectiveness of care. There has been a dramatic increase in the availability of research-based information. Systematic reviews of research reports, the development of programs for assessing health technology, and the rapid development of information and communication technologies have been major contributors to this. While new World Wide Web sites continue to appear, the following are electronic resources available at the time of writing that are likely to prove useful.

1. The Cochrane Collaboration and Library

http://som.flinders.edu.au/FUSA/cochrane/cochrane/general.htm
http://www.update-software.com/ccweb/cochrane/cdsr.htm

The Cochrane Collaboration is an international organization that aims to assist medical decision making by preparing, maintaining, and ensuring the accessibility of systematic reviews of the effects of health care interventions. It has built on methods that were initially used to prepare and maintain reviews of controlled trials of care in pregnancy and childbirth, and it now facilitates systematic reviews of randomized, controlled trials across all areas of health care. The Cochrane Collaboration has evolved rapidly and internationally since it was inaugurated in 1992, but its basic objectives and principles have remained the same as they were at its inception. The United Kingdom focus of the Cochrane Collaboration—the United Kingdom Cochrane Centre at Oxford—is supported under the National Health Service (NHS) Research and Development (R&D) Programme.

The Cochrane Library is an electronic publication covering all areas of health care, designed to supply high quality evidence to inform people about effective health care practices. It is published quarterly on CD-ROM, and includes the Cochrane Database of Systematic Reviews; the Database of Abstracts of Reviews of Effectiveness; the Cochrane Controlled Trials Register (giving brief details of more than 170 000 randomized, controlled trials); and other sources of information on the science of review research and evidence-based health care.

2. Effective Healthcare Bulletins and Effectiveness Matters

http://www.york.ac.uk/inst/crd/ehcb.htm
http://www.york.ac.uk/inst/crd/em.htm

The United Kingdom National Health Service Centre for Reviews and Dissemination (CRD) was established in 1994 to provide the NHS with information on the effectiveness of treatments and the delivery and organization of health care. Within the NHS R&D programme, the CRD is the sibling organization of the United Kingdom Cochrane Centre.

Effectiveness Matters publications are also produced by the CRD. They give information on the effectiveness of important health interventions for practitioners and decision makers. They cover topics in a shorter and more journalistic style, summarizing the results of high quality, systematic reviews.

3. The Oxford Centre for Evidence-Based Medicine

http://cebm.jr2.ox.ac.uk

The Oxford Centre is the first of several centres in the United Kingdom established to create an electronic publishing forum for rapid access to evidence on specific interventions.

4. United States National Library of Medicine PubMed

http://www.nlm.nih.gov/databases/freemedl.html

The MEDLINE database of more than 9 million references to publications in 3900 biomedical journals may be accessed free of charge on the World Wide Web. Two Web-based products, PubMed and Internet Grateful Med, provide this access.

5. Evidence Based Medicine

http://www.bmjpg.com/data/ebm.htm

This is published bimonthly and surveys more than 70 international medical journals to identify the key research papers that are scientifically valid and relevant to practice.

6. United Kingdom Health Technology Assessment Programme

http://www.hta.nhs.web.nhs.uk

Health Technology Assessment is the largest single programme of work in the United Kingdom NHS Research and Development Programme. It takes a broad view of the term 'health technology', and covers all interventions including the use of devices, equipment, and drugs, as well as procedures and care, across the whole spectrum of medical, nursing, and health practice.

7. Netting the Evidence A ScHARR Introduction to Evidence Based Practice on the Internet

http://www.shef.ac.uk/~scharr/ir/netting.html

This is a useful site from which to access evidence-based clinical information.

8. The United States Agency for Health Care Policy and Research (AHCPR)

http://www.ahcpr.gov

The AHCPR, established in December 1989 as a part of the US Department of Health and Human Services, is the leading US agency charged with supporting research designed to improve the quality of health care, reduce its cost, and broaden access to essential services. The AHCPR's broad programmes of research bring practical, science-based information to medical practitioners and to consumers and other health-care purchasers. The AHCPR website posts evidence-based clinical guidelines, and a clearing-house of guidelines will be available on the World Wide Web from December 1998.

9. NHS Economic Evaluation Database

http://nhscrd.york.ac.uk/welcome.html

The NHS Economic Evaluation Database is a database of structured abstracts of economic evaluations of health care interventions. Cost–benefit analyses, cost-effectiveness analyses, and cost–utility analyses are identified from a variety of sources and assessed according to set quality criteria. Detailed, structured abstracts are produced.

10. Scottish Intercollegiate Guidelines

http://pc47.cee.hw.ac.uk/sign/

The Scottish Intercollegiate Guidelines Network (SIGN), formed in 1993, aims to improve the effectiveness and efficiency of clinical care for patients in Scotland by developing, publishing, and disseminating guidelines which identify and promote good clinical practice. SIGN is a network of clinicians and health-care professionals including representatives of all the United Kingdom Royal Medical Colleges as well as nursing, pharmacy, dentistry, and professions allied to medicine. Patients' views are represented on SIGN through the Scottish Association of Health Councils. SIGN works closely with other national groups and government agencies working in the National Health Service in Scotland.

11. The Canadian Taskforce on the Periodic Health Examination

```
http://www.hc-sc.gc.ca/hppb/healthcare/pubs/
clinical_preventive/sec10e.htm
```

The Taskforce's Web site has useful information on clinical preventive services for cancer prevention and control.

1.9 Internet sites for oncologists

Health professionals need to be aware of the resources available on the Internet. It is increasingly common for patients to 'surf the Web' seeking information and clinicians may be presented with printed material down-loaded from various Internet sites. Although there are many Internet sites created by authoritative and reputable bodies (see the selection below), there are also hundreds of other sites relating to cancer with little or no professional or scientific scrutiny, containing information of uncertain validity.

The following is a list of useful Internet sites for oncology health professionals:

- The American Cancer Society homepage
  `http://www.cancer.org/main.html`

- CancerNet
  `http://cancernet.nci.nih.gov/`
  (Maintained by the American National Cancer Institute) is a very useful site for information on specific tumours, 'state of the art' treatment summarized by experts, and lists of active clinical trials in oncology sorted by tumour site. A particularly useful section is a critical and authoritative review of the data on 'alternative' and/or 'unproven' cancer therapies.

- The American Society of Clinical Oncology online
  `http://www.asco.org/`

- State of the Art Oncology in Europe ('StArt')
  `http://telescan.nki.nl/start/`
  This is conducted by the European School of Oncology, providing a database on treatment of tumours, written and reviewed by expert clinicians.

- HealthGate
  `http://www.healthgate.com/`
  This is a site providing general medical information and free access to MEDLINE and other databases.
- World Health Organization
  `http://www.who.org/`
- Medscape
  `http://www.medscape.com/`
  This is another useful site containing meeting reports and abstracts, oncology news, and free searching of MEDLINE.
- Other websites with useful listings and data concerning unproven cancer therapies are:
  `http://www.bccancer.bc/uctm`
  `http://www.sph.uth.tmc.edu/utcam`
- OncoWeb
  `http://www.oncoweb.com/conferences/index.html`

This provides a comprehensive list of upcoming oncology conferences.

1.10 How can one justify a screening programme for cancer?

Many symptomatic cancers affecting humans result in the majority of those afflicted dying as a result of the disease when earlier detection of the cancer may have resulted in cure. As the population life expectancy increases, the prevalence of many age-related cancers also increases as does the attributable risk of cancers to society. The intuitive reflex of the positivist medical practitioner is to embark on early detection of these common cancers with the hope that many lives can be saved and that no cost is too great to save one life. However, clinical practice is becoming more and more resource limited and justification of new practices such as population screening is mandatory. How do we decide to commence screening for such common cancers as colorectal, breast, cervical, prostate, lung, and skin cancers? Why not screen for other less common cancers such as oesophageal, gastric, pancreatic, ovarian, and endometrial to name just a few? Should an asymptomatic 50-year-old female have a mammogram, colonoscopy, pap smear, chest radiograph, and pelvic ultrasound? If so, how often, what other cancers should be included, where do we start and when do we stop?

In assessing screening programmes a logical and methodical stepwise approach is advisable. Firstly, does the cancer in question have a predictable natural history with identifiable stages along the way that lends itself to alteration by screening interventions? These critical points may be the detection and removal of benign precursor lesions (e.g. polyps) or the possibility of earlier detection of better prognostic cancers (e.g. cervical, breast, and bowel). There must be an intervention that is likely to cure the disease for screening to be worthwhile (less likely with cancers such as pancreatic and oesophageal). Other cancers may be so indolent that many will die from other causes despite the presence of cancer. Interventions for these indolent cancers may be more life threatening than the cancer itself (e.g. many cases of prostate cancer).

Once a cancer has been determined to be of significant prevalence combined with a significant population mortality (attributable risk of a cancer) with a potentially curative intervention that is effective, screening can be considered. Step one is to determine the efficacy of the screening test in an ideal setting. The sensitivity, specificity, and cancer detection rates are some indirect measures of the efficacy of a screening manoeuvre but cancer-specific mortality is the most robust measure of efficacy. Overall population survival benefits are less important in this assessment as cancer mortality is dwarfed by the greater effects of cardiovascular mortality. Step two requires the assessment of proven efficacious screening measures (in trials) in the general population (effectiveness). Compliance of the population screened, health professionals, and health providers, together with the perceived and real adverse effects of screening on physical and psychological well being of the population, are integral aspects of this assessment. Step 3 assesses the cost-effectiveness of proven effective screening manoeuvres, often adopting comparative cost per life year saved assessments. The final step is to assess the validity of commencing a proven cost-effective screening manoeuvre. The clinical and the statistical significance of the mortality benefit needs to be evaluated in the context of comparable preventive and therapeutic interventions with the allocation of limited health resources. Differing societies may embrace or reject the same cost–benefit of a cancer screening test.

1.11 Tumour staging

Humans tend to seek patterns in complexity, and to describe and classify that which they hope to understand, and ultimately control.

Tumour staging systems have evolved from an appreciation of the natural history of individual cancers. As understanding of tumour behaviour, and more recently tumour biology, has increased, staging systems have become more complex.

Staging systems have benefits, limitations, and risks.

Individuals benefit from staging systems because such systems help physicians select an appropriate treatment, based upon the experience of others with a similar problem. This may take the form of a treatment guideline. On another level, staging systems suggest questions for further research.

The observation that not all tumours of a particular stage behave the same way begs an explanation. Although partial explanations have been found in tumour biology, staging systems will always lag behind the current level of understanding of a particular tumour type because they have an inherent inertia resulting from their co-operative nature and the rapid rate of progress in biology. Modern staging systems anticipate this lag phenomenon, and it is likely that this increased understanding of malignancy will be reflected eventually in more sophisticated staging systems.

Staging systems allow clinicians to compare groups of patients and to compare different treatments. This aim is idealistic, and unfortunately not always achieved. Different research groups may not agree on which staging system to adopt. Even if agreement is attained, there may be a disparity in the way patients are sorted into a particular stage. The concept of staging is sound, but it is important to be aware of these limitations.

There is no doubt that models derived from staging have advanced our understanding and improved management. However, on a philosophical level, classification can also be a potentially dangerous oversimplification. To take an extreme example, an individual tumour does not 'know' what stage it is. Description can potentially be mistaken for control, or the illusion of control.

Staging systems may carry a more subtle danger by implying a particular mechanism and natural history of disease. A given tumour can only be classified in the terms accepted under a given system. A tumour thus described will confirm and validate the system. The model can become embedded, and can potentially delay the adoption of new concepts for management of a disease.

Tumour staging is a highly successful manifestation of the reductionist philosophy. This may, in part, explain the apparent paradox of its success. While staging systems can accurately predict survival patterns for entire populations of patients with a particular stage of a particular cancer type, we must remind ourselves that this is of little use to the individual faced with the fact that he/she has a 50 per cent chance of surviving 5 years. Maybe they will survive, maybe they will not!

References

1.1
Cobleigh, M., Vogel, C.L., Tripathy, D. *et al.* (1998). Efficacy and safety of humanized anti-HER2 antibody as a single agent in 222 women with HER2 overexpression who relapsed following chemotherapy for metastatic breast cancer. *Proceedings of the American Society for Clinical Oncology*, **17,** (abstract 376).
Kinzler, K.W. and Vogelstein, B. (1996). Lessons from hereditary colorectal cancer. *Cell*, **87**, 159–170.
Matthay, K.K., Perez, C., Seeger, R.C. *et al.* (1998). Successful treatment of stage III neuroblastoma based on prospective biologic staging: a Children's Cancer Group study. *Journal of Clinical Oncology*, **16**, 1256–64.

Pulciani, S., Santos, E., Lauver, A.V., Long, L.K., Aaronson, S.A. and Barbacid, M. (1982). Oncogenes in solid human tumours. *Nature*, **300**, 539–542.

Slamon, D., Leyland-Jones, B., Shack, S. *et al.* (1998). Addition of humanized anti-HER2 antibody to first line chemotherapy for HER2 overexpressing metastatic breast cancer markedly increases anticancer activity. *Proceedings of the American Society for Clinical Oncology*, 17, (abstract 377).

1.2

Kinzler, K.W. and Vogelstein, B. (1998). Landscaping the cancer terrain. *Science*, **280**, 1036–1037.

1.4

Bellamy, C.O. (1997). p53 and apoptosis. *British Medical Bulletin*, **53**, 522–538.

Jansen, B., Schlagbauer-Wadl, H., Brown, B.D. (1998). bcl-2 antisense therapy chemosensitizes human melanoma in SCID mice. *Nature Medicine*, **4**, 232–234.

Newton, K., Strasser, A. (1998). The Bcl-2 family and cell death regulation. *Current Opinions in Genetic Development*, **8**, 68–75.

Takaoka, A., Adachi, M., Okuda, H., *et al.* (1997). Anti-cell death activity promotes pulmonary metastasis of melanoma cells. *Oncogene*, **14**, 2971–2977.

1.5

Baar, J. and Tannock, I. (1989). Analyzing the same data in two ways: a demonstration model to illustrate the reporting and misreporting of clinical trials. *Journal of Clinical Oncology*, 7, 969–978.

Feinstein, A.R., Sosin, D.M., and Wells, C.K. (1985). The Will Rogers phenomenon. Stage migration and new diagnostic techniques as a source of misleading statistics for survival in cancer. *New England Journal of Medicine*, **312**, 1604–1608.

1.6

Anderson, J.R., Cain, K.C., and Gelber, R.D. (1983). Analysis of survival by tumour response. *Journal of Clinical Oncology*, **1**, 710–719.

1.7

Drummond, M.F., O'Brien, B., Stoddart, G.L. and Torrance, G.W. (1997). *Methods for the economic evaluation of health care programs* (2nd edn). Oxford University Press.

Smith, R.D., Hall, J., Gurney, H., and Harnett, P.R. (1993). A cost-utility approach to the use of 5-fluorouracil and levamisole as adjuvant chemotherapy for Dukes 'C' colonic carcinoma. *Medical Journal of Australia*, **158**, 319–322.

1.10

Hunt, J.A. and Solomon, M.J. (1995). Screening for cancer: the science behind the rhetoric. *International Journal of Surgical Science*, **2**, 161–167.

Wilson, J.M.G. and Junger, G. (1968). *Principles and practice of screening for disease*. WHO (Public Health Paper): Geneva.

Making management decisions

2.1 A 34-year-old woman with a cervical lesion

A 34-year-old woman undergoes colposcopy after an abnormal PAP smear reported abnormal cells consistent with cervical intraepithelial neoplasia (CIN) III. At colposcopy there is a 2 cm aceto-white lesion on the ectocervix, the lesion extends inside the canal.

How would you manage this patient?
The principles employed in managing this case are fundamental to the practice of oncology. At this stage of the problem, the decision-making principles are:

* establish the nature of the lesion;
* establish the extent of the lesion;
* understand the natural history of the disease in question.

The nature of the lesion is not yet established. From the colposcopic appearance it is likely that the diagnosis is CIN, but as the entire lesion has not been visualized, it could be microinvasive carcinoma, deeply invasive carcinoma, or possibly an unexpected rarer diagnosis. The diagnostic possibilities therefore include a small limited area of CIN, eminently treatable by local measures, up to and including an invasive cervical carcinoma requiring more radical treatment. A punch biopsy would be insufficient, as the histological information obtained from one part of the lesion may not be completely representative of the remainder of the lesion. On the other hand, a hysterectomy at this stage would be overtreatment for an early CIN lesion.

The appropriate management is cone biopsy which will be diagnostic and a potentially curative therapeutic manoeuvre.

Cone biopsy is performed. The histology report is 'The lesion is predominantly CIN III, but with one area of focal invasion extending 2 mm into the stroma of the cervix'.

What would you do now?
The standard oncological principles to be applied here are:

- establish the extent of the lesion;
- understand the natural history of this disease.

If the margins are clear (note that this has not been stated in the report and should be checked in discussion with the pathologist), and the tumour is only minimally invasive, this lesion would be consistent with a diagnosis of microinvasive carcinoma of the cervix. An understanding of the natural history of this lesion is required to define appropriate management. The likelihood of metastases to regional lymph nodes or beyond is zero in such a case, and treatment can be regarded as complete if margins are clear. If we had embarked upon a hysterectomy when the patient was first seen, we may have overtreated this patient. In a 34-year-old patient, the question of preservation of fertility may be important and therefore hysterectomy may have caused unnecessary loss of fertility when a fertility-sparing cone biopsy may have been adequate.

The pathology report for the same patient may have said: 'The lesion is predominantly CIN III, but there is a focus of squamous cell carcinoma extending 3 mm into the stroma of the cervix. Tumour extends to the excision margin'.

How would you manage this case?
With this histology report it is evident that we have not satisfied the requirements set out earlier. The extent of the tumour has not been defined because the margins of excision are positive. The tumour is most likely worse than *microinvasive* disease with potential for metastases and the need for more radical treatment. Further staging and therapy is required, which could take the form of either hysterectomy or radical irradiation. This raises the next important principle in the management of cancer:

- understand the potential benefits and limitations of surgery, radiation, and chemotherapy for this particular problem.

The design of the management plan needs to take into account the site of disease, patterns of spread, and the effectiveness of various treatment modalities (surgery, radiation therapy, and chemotherapy in this case).

In theory, surgery could be limited to the cervix, involve a simple hysterectomy, or a radical hysterectomy (removing parametrial tissue as well), with or without removal of regional lymph nodes. The best surgical approach will be determined by an understanding of the natural history of the tumour (in other words its patterns of spread and its propensity to spread), and the extent of disease present, for this particular patient. Surgery involving radical hysterectomy and pelvic lymph node dissection offers an 85 per cent 5-year survival for Stage 1B (this patient's likely stage) carcinoma of the cervix.

By the same token, pelvic irradiation including treatment directed at the primary tumour site and regional lymph nodes is equally likely to cure this patient's tumour. The extent of the field would again be defined by understanding the natural history of this tumour.

Chemotherapy, however, has not been shown to be effective in treating such tumours, so is not included amongst the treatment options.

This raises the next important point:

- plan appropriate treatment for *THIS* patient's disease.

Either surgery (as radical hysterectomy and pelvic node dissection) *or* radical pelvic irradiation would have an equal likelihood of curing this tumour. However, one modality may be preferred over another in a particular patient. For example whilst both treatments will have the same negative impact on fertility, surgery allows the potential for preservation of the ovaries, whereas radical pelvic irradiation will inevitably result in the patient becoming menopausal at a very young age. Sexual function after surgery is also likely to be more satisfactory than after radiation therapy. Hence in most young patients and indeed older patients with early disease (confined to the cervix) radical hysterectomy is the preferred treatment.

In a patient who is medically unsuitable for anaesthesia, irradiation may be the more appropriate modality.

New approaches to therapy such as radical trachelectomy (radical resection of the cervix with preservation of the uterine fundus) and lymph node dissection may be acceptable. A younger patient, after discussion of the potential risks and uncertainties of such a novel approach, may choose this controversial but fertility-sparing treatment.

The patient undergoes radical hysterectomy and pelvic lymph node dissection. At surgery, several of the pelvic lymph nodes are noted to be hard and enlarged. Nine out of 23 regional lymph nodes contain metastatic squamous cell carcinoma. There is extra capsular spread of tumour from two of these lymph nodes.

How would you manage this patient now?
Again, understanding the natural history of the disease is important in guiding management. There is a significant potential for local recurrence, despite the surgery. Moreover the presence of extensive metastatic disease

within the lymph nodes indicates the metastatic potential of this particular tumour, and signifies a relatively high risk of distant metastases.

It would be appropriate to consider pelvic irradiation, which would reduce the likelihood of pelvic recurrence. Pelvic irradiation however will have no effect on ultimate survival, as it leaves more distant metastases untreated. The addition of pelvic irradiation after surgical lymphadenectomy significantly increases the likelihood of morbidity including troublesome leg lymphoedema, bowel injury, and bladder dysfunction, and this would require careful discussion with the patient. The risk of adverse effects should be weighed against the risk of pelvic tumour recurrence. Many decisions in oncology require such balanced assessments of competing risks.

The patient wishes to think this decision over for a few days. One week later she returns for a scheduled visit and brings with her a printout of an article downloaded from the Internet. The article describes the beneficial effects of chemotherapy for breast cancer which has spread to regional lymph nodes. She asks whether she should have chemotherapy.

How would you answer her?
Such requests are best answered by discussing available evidence as it applies to this particular patient. In a number of tumour types (e.g. breast, colon carcinoma), adjuvant chemotherapy provides modest improvements in recurrence rates and survival. There is no conclusive evidence that adjuvant systemic therapy improves the outcome of high-risk *cervical* carcinoma. However, this is not the same as saying 'there is evidence that adjuvant systemic therapy does *not* improve the outcome'. The balanced view would therefore be that adjuvant systemic therapy *may* ultimately prove to be of benefit, but should not be recommended as standard therapy.

The patient may wish to enrol in a well-designed, prospective clinical trial investigating the role of adjuvant systemic therapy. Such studies are essential to advance knowledge and perhaps improve therapy.

Clinicians considering a potential clinical trial have several obligations; the clinician must be sure that the trial addresses a valid question, that the treatment arms of the study are all reasonable therapy 'in equipoise', and that the trial is designed and conducted so that an answer to the question will indeed be obtained (that is the trial will accrue sufficient patients to have the statistical power to confirm or exclude an effect of the new therapy with reasonable statistical certainty).

Patients must give informed consent before participation. Many patients are prepared to consider participation in clinical trials, as long as the toxicity of the new treatment appears reasonable, and they are sure that the doctor believes that whatever treatment they might receive on trial will be a good treatment option for them as an individual. Moreover, there is good evidence that patients who are treated on clinical trials have a better outcome than the non-trial population. The reasons why are not entirely clear, but probably include selection bias and the benefit of the relatively intense follow-up and supportive care inherent in the conduct of clinical research practice.

2.2 Assessing the benefits of adjuvant therapies

A previously well, 61-year-old man has recently undergone a left hemicolectomy for colon cancer situated distal to the splenic flexure. He has made a good post-operative recovery and has no significant past medical or family history. A pre-operative CT scan of the abdomen and pelvis showed no evidence of distant disease. Pathology showed a moderately differentiated adenocarcinoma, extending through the muscularis to the pericolic fat. None of 12 lymph nodes had evidence of malignant infiltration ($T_2N_0M_0$) or Dukes' B_2. At the suggestion of his surgeon, he asks your advice about adjuvant chemotherapy.

How do you assess the indications for adjuvant therapy?
The main questions we wish to answer here are whether adjuvant therapy will improve disease-free survival or overall survival, by how much, and whether any such improvement is worth the toxicity of treatment.

Randomized trials of adjuvant chemotherapy for colon cancer have been carried out for decades. Most experts suggest focusing on studies published from about 1990 onwards, since this is when adequate doses and duration of treatment were used in moderate to large-scale trials. Several trials of 5-fluorouracil based adjuvant chemotherapy show a reduction in the risk of recurrence and death for patients with localized colon cancer. Thus the biological principle that adjuvant treatment prevents (or delays) colon cancer recurrence appears secure.

These trials enrolled patients with both node-positive and node-negative disease, the node negative disease being T_3 (Dukes' B_2). Overall, the *risk of recurrence* is reduced by about a third and death by a fifth. There is no good reason why effect should be substantially different in different stages of disease, and certainly the very extensively validated breast cancer literature convincingly shows the same *proportional* effects of treatment in both node-negative and node-positive tumours. Thus the key question is what are the *absolute benefits* of treatment?

For node-positive patients (Dukes' C disease) the risk of death is high—at least 50 per cent—and thus reducing a 50 per cent risk of death by one fifth is quite substantial. Although results vary somewhat between studies (as to doses, duration, and drugs used), there is probably at least a 10 per cent absolute difference in survival rates at 10 years.

For node-negative ($T_3 N_0$) (Dukes' B_2) disease, the risk of death is much lower (only about 15 per cent in this case in some studies), so there is much less absolute benefit to gain. Absolute survival benefits are likely to be a few percentage points only.

To return to this patient, he needs to know that some schedule of adjuvant chemotherapy (most likely involving 5 FU and folinic acid and lasting about 6 months) would change his chances of being alive at 5 years from perhaps 85 per cent to perhaps 88 or 89 per cent. Mild to moderate toxicity would be involved (frequent clinic visits, mild nausea, mouth ulcers, and diarrhoea for perhaps 2 or 3 days a month).

As the breast cancer experience shows, fashions change. In the late 1990s, most patients with $T_3 N_0$ colon cancer in Britain and Australia would be strongly urged to have adjuvant chemotherapy, though many would in the United States. There is thus still considerable room for discussion with patients about personal preferences.

The patient who says, 'I want everything that could possibly help my chances' should have chemotherapy.

The patient who says, 'I'm scared of needles' probably should not.

2.3 A 73-year-old woman with a bone lesion

A 73-year-old woman, who has been in good health all her life, presents with discomfort in the right groin on weight bearing. You do a radiograph of the pelvis which is reported as follows: 'There is an area of bone lysis with irregular thinning of the cortex in the upper third of the right femur, highly suggestive of metastasis.'

How would you manage this patient?
As in the first case, the nature of the lesion must be established. Even though most such cases will indeed be due to malignant disease, all experienced clinicians can recount cases of benign or other unexpected pathology presenting with so-called 'typical' features of malignancy. It is a sound working principle that:

- cancer is a diagnosis which is reached ONLY by obtaining a tissue diagnosis, not by radiological or clinical features alone.

Although occasional circumstances arise where the clinical scenario is such that a tissue diagnosis is thought unnecessary or even meddlesome, the prudent clinician thinks carefully before abandoning a tissue diagnosis.

A standard history and systems review is vital, including specific questioning on previous, sometimes forgotten or disregarded, episodes such as removal of supposedly benign skin lesions (which may in fact have been malignant). Physical examination should include rectal and vaginal examination, careful assessment of the entire skin surface, and urinalysis. A plain chest radiograph should be obtained. Disorders which may be diagnosed on blood test (e.g. myeloma, hypercalcaemia, etc.) should be considered. Any abnormalities detected are then followed through as appropriate to establish a tissue diagnosis.

If no abnormalities are detected, a tissue diagnosis from the bone lesion is even more relevant. An orthopaedic procedure could both obtain a tissue diagnosis and treat the bone lesion.

The options for therapy for the local bone lesion include irradiation of the lesion to prevent progressive bone loss leading to further pain and ultimately pathological fracture. If the bone is already significantly weakened (i.e. more than one-third of the cortical bone thickness is lost), prophylactic orthopaedic fixation should be considered prior to irradiation.

The most common tissue diagnosis in this setting is metastatic carcinoma (often adenocarcinoma) from an unknown primary tumour. Investigations beyond those described above are unlikely to detect a primary tumour. Mammograms and CT scans are unlikely to be helpful. Moreover, in the uncommon event that an otherwise occult primary tumour is detected by such investigations, this is unlikely to help determine management as the tumour is already beyond cure by surgery, and the prognosis is poor (median of 4 months).

There are exceptions to this rule however:

- patients presenting with neck nodes containing squamous cell carcinoma (which may represent an occult primary in the head and neck);
- females presenting with axillary adenopathy containing adenocarcinoma (which often represents occult breast cancer);
- females presenting with ascites and peritoneal carcinomatosis, which often represents occult ovarian/primary peritoneal carcinoma;
- males presenting with a midline distribution (i.e. para-aortic/mediastinal pattern) lymphadenopathy which may represent an extragonadal germ cell tumour.

These exceptional circumstances should be managed along lines appropriate for their presumptive primary tumour, with similar prognosis.

These syndromes aside, chemotherapy is of limited value in the syndrome of metastatic carcinoma *unknown primary* (CUP) which is the most likely diagnosis in this case. Response rates are around 20 per cent, and response durations typically short. Chemotherapy is probably best reserved for palliation of symptoms which are difficult to manage by other means. Such symptoms may sometimes include the patient's (or families') view that 'we can't just sit back and let the cancer grow!' Although entirely understandable, this reaction, or the more commonly put view that 'there is nothing to lose', is in many cases incorrect. For CUP patients with minimal or easily controlled symptoms, the use of toxic therapies is likely to reduce quality of life. Given a response rate of only 20 per cent in the face of a short survival time, many patients are worse off from such treatment. A gentle but truthful discussion of these issues with the patient and family will assist good decision making.

It is an important principle of all medicine that:

- the goal of treatment determines the form of treatment.

If cure were a realistic goal, then considerable short-term toxicity might be appropriate in order to achieve the goal of cure. If therapy could prolong survival, then a certain degree of toxicity might be worthwhile when traded-off against the length of lifetime gained. However, if treatment will not cure, or even prolong survival, it is important to monitor the balance between toxicity and benefit. Merely exchanging symptoms from cancer for toxicity of treatment is clearly inappropriate.

The humane aspect of management is just as important as the technical aspect. Until a tissue diagnosis is reached, no diagnosis or prognosis can or should be given to the patient, no matter how 'typical' the clinical pattern. When bad news is suspected, most patients do best when a range of diagnostic possibilities is mentioned at the outset, including the possibility of malignancy, amongst others. Bad news broken into instalments as test results come in sequentially can be an effective strategy. The principle is not to delude, but to assist with staged assimilation of a major life event.

The patient's own goals, attitudes, and general health are all of relevance in making management decisions. A socially isolated patient may approach this problem differently to a patient eagerly awaiting the marriage of a child or the birth of a grandchild. Such short-term goals can exert major influence on treatment decisions in oncology, as can the existence of significant comorbidities (e.g. diabetes, vascular disease, etc.).

The principles of decision making in oncology are:
- establish the nature of the lesion—cancer is a diagnosis reached only by obtaining a tissue diagnosis, not by radiological or clinical features alone;
- establish the extent of the tumour;
- understand the natural history of the tumour;
- understand the potential benefits and limitations of surgery, radiation, and chemotherapy for treatment of this tumour;
- plan treatment appropriate for the specific needs of the individual patient;
- understand the role of clinical trials in improving cancer care.

2.4 Human error

A 2nd year resident miscalculates a dose of chemotherapy, potentially resulting in a ten-fold overdose.

'To err is human' yet many parts of society (including hospitals) rely completely on error free performance. Error is associated with shame, guilt, and other unpleasant negative emotions and it follows that a person who has made an error does not usually want to talk about it. Valuable information about how to avoid errors is lost because people who have made the error keep it to themselves. High technology industries, such as aviation, have successful methods of coping with the reality of human error. These modern industries extract the greatest possible information from errors and use this information to build a successful and safe industry. Unfortunately, medicine has become a high technology industry with an internal culture that denies human error. The understandable need of patients to feel (to 'know') that their doctor is infallible reinforces this paradigm. As a result, the profession is poorly equipped to manage the reality of mistakes as they occur (and they occur often).

In this case, the miscalculation is picked up by an experienced nurse before the drug is given. The resident becomes preoccupied by his mistake and worries about what would have happened if a less experienced nurse, unfamiliar with the field, had given the drug at the dose he ordered. He becomes depressed and wonders if he has chosen a career for which he is unsuited.

A system that is designed around the reality of human performance considers the causes of error (which can be multifactorial), how to prevent further similar errors, and the effect that having made the error has on the protagonist.

The resident is formally debriefed by one of the senior consultants and comes to realize that he is not the only doctor to have made an error. He reads the definitive article by Lucian Leape and other work by cognitive psychologist, James Reason and realizes that the error was the result of a complex set of circumstances; he was new on the unit having just returned from secondment to a country term. He was ordering a new drug of which he had no experience. He had worked the previous nightshift for a colleague and had spent the last 27 hours on duty. He was concerned because he had done little study toward his professional exams which were coming up in 2 weeks.

The unit institutes a more formal drug checking mechanism but most of the underlying factors referred to in the last paragraph remain unaddressed.

One of the problems with coming to terms with this issue is the fact that the community is not prepared to acknowledge that human factors influence their physicians. Some sectors of the community rely for their living on error, imperfect performance, and the misleading (and overly simplistic) concepts of blame and negligence. This short-sighted approach makes it even more difficult for this problem to be discussed openly. The aviation industry delivers safe transportation against extraordinary odds by adopting a realistic approach to the limitations of human performance; medicine could do the same.

References

2.2

IMPACT Investigators (1995). Efficacy of adjuvant fluorouracil and folinic acid in colon cancer. *Lancet*, **345**, 939–944.

Moertel, C.G., Fleming, T.R., Macdonald, J.S. *et al.* (1995). Fluorouracil plus levamisole as effective adjuvant therapy after resection of stage III colon carcinoma: a final report. *Annals of Internal Medicine*, **122**, 321–326.

O'Connell, M.J., Laurie, J.A., Kahn, M. *et al.* (1998). Prospectively randomized trial of postoperative adjuvant chemotherapy in patients with high-risk colon cancer. *Journal of Clinical Oncology*, **16,** 295–300.

2.4

Leape, L.L. (1994). Error in medicine. *Journal of the American Medical Association*, **272**, 1851–1857.

Reason, J. (1992). *Human error*. Cambridge University Press: Cambridge, Mass.

Breast oncology

3.1 How does family history define increased risk of breast cancer?

In Australia, 1 in 11 women will develop breast cancer over their lifetime.

A 30-year-old woman, Janet, attends your surgery. She has two young children. Her previous health has been excellent. She has read that a family history of breast cancer may influence her own risk of breast cancer.

For each of the following situations, look at the family tree and estimate the level of risk for Janet according to the family history.

In the first case (Fig. 3.1), Janet has one first-degree relative with breast cancer at age 60. Reassure Janet that her risk is at or slightly above average for the general population and that about 90 per cent of women with this history will not get breast cancer.

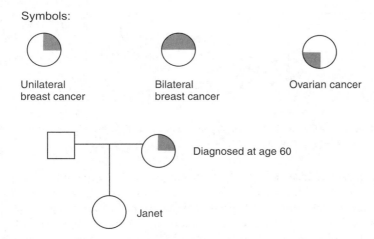

Fig. 3.1 Family tree for case 1—one first-degree affected relative.

In the second case (Fig. 3.2), Janet has one first-degree and one second-degree relative with breast cancer, diagnosed at ages 60 and 73, *but* they are on different sides of the family. Reassure Janet that she is at or slightly above average for the general population and that about 90 per cent of women with this history will not get breast cancer.

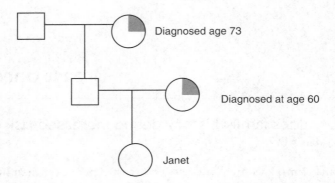

Fig. 3.2 Family tree for case 2—one first-degree and one second-degree affected relative. Symbols as in Fig. 3.1.

In the third case (Fig. 3.3), Janet has one first-degree and one second-degree relative with breast cancer, diagnosed at ages 53 and 57, *and* they are on the same side of the family. Advise Janet that she has a moderately increased risk of developing breast cancer (lifetime risk 1 in 8 to 1 in 4), but 70 to 90 per cent of women in this group will not get breast cancer.

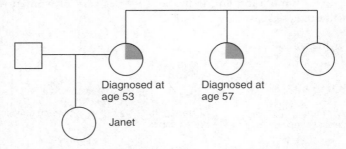

Fig. 3.3 Family tree for case 3—one first-degree and one second-degree affected relative on the same side of the family. Symbols as in Fig. 3.1.

In the fourth case (Fig. 3.4), Janet has one first-degree and one second-degree relative with *early-onset* breast cancer, on the same side of the family. Less than 5 per cent of all breast cancer is due to a strong genetic predisposition. There is a reasonable chance that the women with breast cancer in this family carry a dominantly inherited germline mutation in a breast cancer susceptibility gene, such as *BRCA1* or *BRCA2*. Approximately 1 in 800 individuals carry such a mutation (1 in 50 to 100 Ashkenazi Jewish individuals). Females who carry a mutation in *BRCA1* or *BRCA2* are at increased risk of breast and ovarian cancer. Males who carry a mutation in either gene are at some increased risk of prostate cancer. Germline *BRCA2* mutations also predispose to male breast cancer. Such mutations are inherited in a dominant manner. This history means that Janet is at

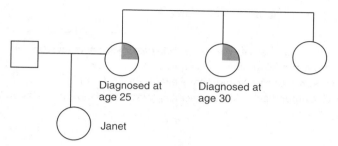

Fig. 3.4 Family tree for case 4—one first-degree and one second-degree affected relative with early-onset breast cancer, on the same side of the family. Symbols as in Fig. 3.1.

potentially high risk, since there is a 50–50 chance that she has inherited a high-risk mutation from her mother, if a mutation is present. Janet's lifetime risk of breast cancer is 1 in 4 to 1 in 2, or higher if she is shown to have a high-risk breast cancer gene mutation.

This time (Fig. 3.5), the history of breast cancer is on Janet's father's side of the family. The paternal history is just as important as the maternal side. This family has four women with breast/ovarian cancer in three generations. The family shows the features of a dominantly inherited breast/ovarian cancer predisposition, which may be due to a mutation in a gene such as *BRCA1* or *BRCA2*.

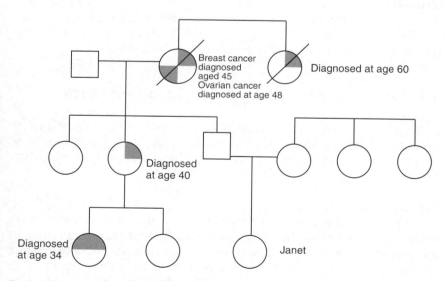

Fig. 3.5 Family tree for case 5—affected relatives on the father's side of the family. Symbols as in Fig. 3.1.

The important features to note are:

- there are a number of women with breast/ovarian cancer on the same side of the family, in different generations;
- at least some of the women have early-onset cancer;
- several women have multiple primary cancers (breast and ovarian cancer/bilateral breast cancer).

As in the fourth case, Janet is at potentially high risk and referral to a specialized familial cancer service is appropriate for risk assessment, advice regarding early detection/prevention of cancer, genetic counselling, and consideration of genetic testing to clarify risk.

The key to assessing risk of cancer due to family history is to take an accurate, extended, two to three generation pedigree documenting all individuals, both with and without cancer, on *both sides* of the family. The type of cancer and the age of onset is important. Overall, less than 5 per cent of all cancer is due to the presence of a dominantly inherited gene mutation which results in a significantly increased risk of cancer in those family members who carry the gene mutation. Specialized familial cancer services have been developed for genetic counselling and genetic testing of such families, if appropriate.

'Current Best Advice about Familial Aspects of Breast Cancer' is the guidelines prepared by the Genetic Testing Working Group of the NHMRC National Breast Cancer Centre (NBCC). This document and a list of specialist genetic services for breast cancer are available through the National Breast Cancer Centre, P O Box 572, Kings Cross NSW 2011, Australia. Telephone: (02) 9334 1700, Fax: (02) 9326 9329.

3.2 Tamoxifen chemoprevention for breast cancer

A 42-year-old woman inquires about taking tamoxifen as chemoprevention for breast cancer. Her mother and one sister have been treated for breast cancer, and her grandmother recently died of ovarian cancer. The patient herself is well, with no breast symptoms.

How would you advise her?
There is Level 1 evidence that tamoxifen given as adjuvant treatment for breast cancer reduces the incidence of contralateral primary tumours. This observation led to the instigation of several clinical trials of tamoxifen as a chemopreventive agent for breast cancer. Results from three randomized, placebo-controlled trials of tamoxifen (20 mg daily) have been reported. In the largest of these, (NSABP Protocol P1) daily tamoxifen for a mean of 3.5

years reduced the incidence of invasive breast cancer by about 45 per cent in North American women. Tamoxifen use also reduced the incidence of ductal carcinoma *in situ* and osteoporotic bone fractures. However, tamoxifen use was associated with a dramatic increase in the risk of endometrial carcinoma and venous thrombosis/pulmonary embolism. In sharp contrast, two smaller studies, in British and Italian women, showed no evidence of reduction in breast cancer incidence. Adverse effects of tamoxifen similar to those seen in the American study were noted in these studies.

The reasons for discrepant results from these clinical trials are uncertain. It is of great interest that in the British trial, a high proportion (36 per cent) of participants were likely to have had a genetic (*BRCA1* or *2*) predisposition to breast cancer (see 1.2 and 3.1 above). The negative result from this study raises the possibility that tamoxifen may not prevent breast cancer in the group with the highest degree of risk.

The results from the American trial are potentially of great significance. The magnitude of the observed effect is consistent with the reduction in contralateral primaries seen in adjuvant studies, and also with a similar effect seen in women taking raloxifene (a selective oestrogen response modifier) for osteoporosis. Early data on tumours occurring in participants in this trial suggest, not surprisingly, that tamoxifen predominantly reduces the incidence of oestrogen receptor positive tumours. However, it must be emphasized that no data are available yet to demonstrate that this reduction will translate into improved survival of the patient cohort taking tamoxifen. For example the data available to date would be consistent with several effects:

- that tamoxifen prevents the genesis of tumours;
- that tamoxifen delays, but does not prevent, the ultimate development of primary tumours;
- that tamoxifen has no effect upon development of primary tumours, but suppresses growth of subclinical receptor positive tumours, thus delaying their detection.

Considerably longer follow-up of women on these trials, assessment of overall survival for both trial arms, and for patients who develop breast cancer on study, is required to resolve these issues. In addition, another study (the 'IBIS' trial) continues to accrue participants.

3.3 Breast cancer with extensive intraductal component—is mastectomy necessary?

A 54-year-old woman has an abnormal mammogram showing a 30 mm area of grouped atypical microcalcifications. A needle-localized wide-local excision of this region is performed. Histology confirms an area of infiltrating ductal carcinoma measuring 9 mm with prominent ductal carcinoma *in situ* (DCIS) within the main tumour mass, and areas of DCIS outside the main tumour mass. Margins are negative by 5 mm. A specimen mammogram and postbiopsy mammogram of the tumour site reveal that all microcalcifications have been removed.

What are the treatment options for this patient?
This patient could be adequately treated by radiotherapy to the remaining breast tissue!

Many clinicians have wrongly assumed that the presence of an *e*xtensive *i*ntraduct *c*omponent (EIC+) tumour is an absolute indication for mastectomy. A scheme for management of EIC+ tumours is shown in Fig.3.6.

EIC+ tumours are reported by some (but not all) centres to be

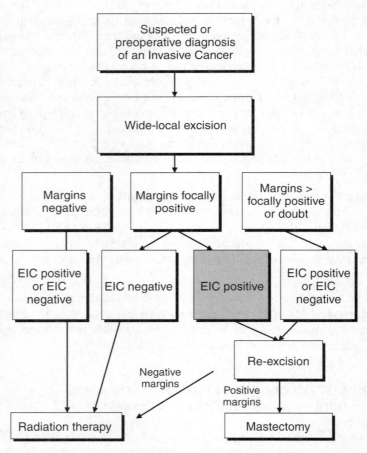

Fig. 3.6 Local management of invasive breast cancer—influence of margins and an extensive intraductal component (EIC). Boyages (1977).

associated with increased risk of a breast cancer recurrence. Differing results from different centres relate, at least in part, to varying definitions of EIC. However, studies with strict criteria for definition of EIC confirm that the main factor predictive of a breast cancer recurrence is an extensive intraductal component (EIC+ tumour).

An EIC+ tumour is defined as:

- the presence of *prominent* intraductal carcinoma within the main tumour mass of an infiltrating ductal cancer and the presence of any intraductal cancer outside the main tumour mass;

or

- predominantly intraductal cancer with one or more areas of focal invasion.

EIC only applies to patients with an infiltrating ductal carcinoma. The presence of lobular carcinoma *in situ* in the presence of an infiltrating ductal or infiltrating lobular carcinoma is not a risk factor for recurrence in the breast after conservative surgery and radiation therapy.

Table 3.1 below shows the probability of a tumour recurrence in the breast based on the presence of the intraductal component within or adjacent to the main tumour mass. Patients with EIC positive tumours are classified as W+A+, while the remainder (W–A–, W–A+, or W+A–) are EIC negative (EIC–)

Table 3.1 Probability of a breast cancer recurrence based on the presence of an intraductal component after conservative surgery and radiation therapy

Intraductal component	Number of patients studied	5-year actuarial local breast cancer relapse (%)
W–A–	138	3
W–A+	141	6
W+A–	23	5
W+A+	143	25

W = within; A = adjacent; + = positive; − = negative

Patients with an EIC+ tumour usually require wider surgery to obtain clear margins than patients with EIC- tumours and are more likely to have a larger residual tumour burden in the remaining breast after a local excision of an infiltrating ductal carcinoma. Patients with an EIC+ tumour and positive or focally positive margins require further surgery (re-excision and perhaps ultimately mastectomy if re-excision shows significant residual disease with involved margins). However, most patients with an EIC+ tumour will achieve a negative re-excision after an initial local excision. In many cases, defining the edge of the invasive tumour is straightforward. However, in some cases, this is more difficult because of the very irregular growth pattern and the stellate shape of carcinoma. A postsurgical mammogram (with magnification views of the excision site) may be helpful when there is doubt about the margins of resection and calcifications are present on a preoperative mammogram.

Once negative margins are achieved, irradiation of the remaining breast tissue is indicated, and this therapeutic approach achieves excellent long-term local control rates.

3.4 Paget's disease of the nipple

A 46-year-old woman presents with a non-healing 'eczema-like' rash measuring 7 mm on the edge of her right nipple, extending to the areola. There is no other abnormality on physical examination and a mammogram is entirely normal. An MRI scan reveals no other evidence of pathology in the retroareolar region, nor the remainder of the breast. The abnormal area is excised, and the histopathology report describes Paget's disease of the nipple with wide areas of Pagetoid cells but no evidence of invasion beyond the basement membrane and no evidence of further disease more proximally in the excised ducts. Immunohistochemical stains for melanoma and squamous cell carcinoma antigens are negative. The lesion has been completely excised with at least a 2-mm margin on the skin surface and a 10-mm margin on the deep surface.

What further management would you advise?
Mastectomy has been the treatment of choice, but increasingly there are reports of success with breast-conserving techniques. These generally involve wide local excision encompassing the nipple and areola complex together with the major ducts and any palpable lump, usually combined with axillary dissection and radiotherapy to the remaining breast tissue.

Paget's disease constitutes around 1 per cent of breast cancer cases. The histogenesis of Paget's cells is now generally thought to be 'epidermotrophic' (i.e. due to underlying tumour cells infiltrating the epidermis). Specialized immunohistochemical stains are helpful in excluding the diagnoses of melanoma or squamous metaplasia/carcinoma. Management issues include:

- distinguishing between benign eczematous rashes versus malignancy;
- the prognostic significance of the presence or absence of an associated mass lesion (median survival 42 months with a mass, and without a mass 126 months).

Recent data suggests that ductal carcinoma *in situ* (DCIS) is frequently the underlying pathology in Paget's disease (Table 3.2).

Magnetic resonance imaging (MRI) is useful in the assessment of the retroareolar region. Use of MRI may improve the limited sensitivity of clinical examination and mammography in finding other underlying

Table 3.2 Pathology and median survival in Paget's disease

Pathology	Mass present	Mass absent
Invasive cancer	75%	36%
Ductal carcinoma *in situ*	57%	64%
Nodal involvement	75%	21%
Median survival (months)	42	126

pathology, including multifocal tumours. A management approach can be formulated if Paget's disease is regarded as adenocarcinoma of the breast presenting at the nipple, but with the special problem that it may be associated with other, deeper lesions that are hard to detect:

- excision biopsy of the nipple lesion;
- if invasive carcinoma is found, or if a mass lesion is detected by examination or imaging (including MRI), then either Patey mastectomy *or* a breast conservation approach employing wide local excision incorporating the nipple, areola, and major ducts together with any mass lesion, axillary dissection, and irradiation of the remaining breast tissue;
- if there is no mass, or the lesion is small (<10 mm), and there is no evidence of further pathology on clinical examination, mammography, ultrasound, or MRI, then observation is appropriate;
- if there is a larger lesion but it is completely excised and there is no evidence of invasion or other lesion, then either Patey mastectomy or a breast conservation protocol is appropriate.

With increasing public awareness of breast cancer it is likely that more cases of Paget's disease will present at an early stage, and should therefore be approached as for any other adenocarcinoma of the breast. Mastectomy should not be regarded as inevitable.

3.5 Should everyone with early breast cancer receive adjuvant radiotherapy?

You receive a referral letter concerning a new patient:

Dear Doctor,

Thank you for seeing this 41-year-old, premenopausal woman with early breast cancer. After noting a right breast lump, she underwent fine needle aspiration biopsy that demonstrated malignancy. She chose to have a mastectomy, and has made a good postoperative recovery. Pathology revealed a 3.5-cm infiltrating ductal carcinoma of grade 3 histology. Immunohistochemical staining for both oestrogen and progesterone receptors was negative. Two of 13 lymph nodes were involved. She has been previously well. Should she have adjuvant radiotherapy?

How would you respond?

There is unequivocal evidence that for patients with early breast cancer, wide local excision of the cancer with irradiation of the remaining breast (i.e. breast conservation therapy) results in survival equivalent to that achieved with mastectomy. Patients with completely excised ductal carcinoma *in situ* also have the choice of breast conservation or mastectomy with equivalent cure rates (see Case 3.3 above).

This woman has already undergone mastectomy. Postmastectomy irradiation reduces the risk of local recurrence after mastectomy. Recent data also suggests that optimizing local control can have an effect on disease-free and overall survival. As holds for adjuvant chemotherapy, postmastectomy radiotherapy is likely to produce a fixed proportional reduction in breast cancer recurrences, but the size of the absolute benefit will be substantially greater for patients with a high risk of recurrence than those with a low risk of recurrence (see Case 2.2 and Case 3.6). Some patients will be at such a low risk of disease recurrence that the burden of therapy will outweigh the benefits.

There is an emerging consensus to recommend postmastectomy radiotherapy for patients with four or more involved axillary nodes, and tumours larger than 5 cm in size (in whom the 5-year risk of locoregional recurrence is around 30 per cent).

By these criteria, the patient described here would not be advised to have postmastectomy radiotherapy.

Many issues require further study and clarification—for example more precise prediction of risk of treatment failure for an individual patient, the extent of the radiotherapy fields (the inclusion of axillary and/or internal mammary nodes), technical advances such as conformal therapy, the scheduling of chemotherapy and radiotherapy (which goes first?), and the potential for enhanced toxicity (both acute and long term) from multi-modality therapy.

3.6 Should everyone with early breast cancer receive adjuvant chemotherapy?

You receive the following referral letter concerning a new patient:

Dear Doctor,

Thank you for seeing this 41-year-old premenopausal woman with early breast cancer. After noting a right breast lump, she underwent fine needle aspiration biopsy that demonstrated malignancy. She proceeded to lumpectomy and axillary dissection and has made a good postoperative recovery. Pathology reveals a 1.5 cm infiltrating ductal carcinoma of grade 3 histology. Immunohistochemical staining for both oestrogen and progesterone receptors is negative. None of 13 lymph nodes are involved. She has been previously well. Should she have adjuvant chemotherapy?

How would you advise her?

Before answering this question, it is worthwhile reviewing the rationale for offering adjuvant treatment. On the basis that certain treatments are known to have an antitumour effect in advanced disease, they are given to patients with early disease in an attempt to reduce the risk of relapse after definitive local therapy. Such an approach has been proven to reduce the risk of relapse and prolong overall survival in breast cancer, colon cancer, and osteogenic sarcoma. Data about other cancers are accumulating.

Adjuvant treatment for early breast cancer may be with chemotherapy, antioestrogens, ovarian ablation (in premenopausal women), or combinations of these. Antioestrogens appear to be ineffective in women with receptor-negative tumours, and should not be considered in this particular case. At least one randomized trial suggests the same is true for ovarian ablation. If adjuvant chemotherapy had no toxicity at all but a small benefit in terms of tumour recurrence and overall survival, then it would be sensible to recommend it to everyone. This of course is not the case. Therefore, as with all medical decisions, the doctor and patient must weigh up risks and benefits based on the available evidence, then apply them to the situation at hand, taking into account patient preferences.

The benefits of adjuvant chemotherapy are best regarded in two distinct ways. In biological terms, chemotherapy will cause a proportional reduction in the risk of tumour recurrence of about a third. This applies to any subset of premenopausal women; in other words the proportional reduction in risk will be about the same whether the tumour is large or small and whether the axillary nodes are positive or negative.

In practical terms however, the absolute risk reduction will depend on the baseline risk. Some over-simplified calculations can help put this into perspective. For example consider a woman with bad prognosis, node-positive disease for whom the disease-free survival at 5 years is 40 per cent. Her risk of recurrence over that time is therefore 60 per cent, and adjuvant chemotherapy will reduce this on average by a third to make it 40 per cent. Her 5-year disease-free survival increases from 40 per cent to 60 per cent, a major benefit that would clearly justify the toxicity of treatment. Conversely, a woman with a very small, node-negative, low grade tumour might have a disease-free survival of 97 per cent. Her risk of recurrence of 3 per cent will be reduced by a third to 2 per cent. Her five year disease-free survival increases from 97 per cent to 98 per cent, a trivial difference which may not be worth 6 months of chemotherapy.

To answer the referring doctor's question, we need to know:

- What is the risk that her tumour will recur over a given period?
- What effect will chemotherapy have on that risk?
- What are the short and long-term side effects of the chemotherapy?

This patient is young and we should therefore be concerned about her long-term outlook. While the chance of a tumour recurrence in the first 5 years is very low, over 10 to 20 years it may approach 20 per cent because the tumour is of grade 3 histology. This could be reduced by a third to about 13 per cent, so her long-term disease-free survival would change from about 80 per cent to about 87 per cent. An element of subjective judgement comes in here of course, for both patient and doctor. Most chemotherapy protocols are reasonably well tolerated, and there is very little evidence of long-term complications, especially for the CMF (cyclophosphamide, methotrexate and 5-fluorouracil) regimen. In the United States, all such women would probably be recommended chemotherapy, while in Canada, the United Kingdom, and Australia many, but not all, oncologists would do the same. With regard to patient preferences, an Australian study (Early Breast Cancer Trialist's Collaborative Group 1998b) demonstrated that many women with breast cancer were prepared to undergo adjuvant chemotherapy for quite small anticipated benefits. Whatever decision is made about chemotherapy, the patient should of course also have radiotherapy, since she had breast-conserving surgery.

3.7 Oophorectomy after breast cancer

A letter from a gynaecologist concerning a patient recently treated for early breast cancer states:

Dear Doctor,

This woman whom you have recently treated for breast cancer requires a hysterectomy for anaemia due to severe intermenstrual bleeding and fibroids. She has read that oophorectomy may prolong survival after breast cancer. She is only 38, and I am uncertain whether this is a good idea. Should she have an oophorectomy at the time of hysterectomy?'

It would be useful to know the oestrogen receptor status of the initial breast cancer, and whether or not the woman received prior adjuvant systemic chemotherapy.

For women with breast cancer under the age of 50, ovarian ablation improves recurrence-free survival (by 6 per cent in absolute terms) and overall survival (by 6.3 per cent in absolute terms) after 15 years of follow-up. The benefits are seen for both node positive and node negative disease. The beneficial effects of ovarian ablation are most evident in patients whose tumours are oestrogen receptor positive, and are probably minimal for patients with oestrogen receptor negative tumours.

One of the concerns about the use of ovarian ablation in young patients is the toxicity. Healthy, young patients who undergo surgical ovarian ablation are expected to develop significant menopausal symptoms within days of ablation and may require hormone supplementation to achieve an acceptable quality of life. The risks and benefits of the use of hormone replacement therapy in patients treated for breast cancer remains controversial. In addition, the standard management of breast cancer with surgery, radiation, and, perhaps, chemotherapy, potentially inflicts quite a significant assault on the femininity and sexuality of the patient. The potential additional effect of adding surgical castration to an already rigorous treatment programme must be considered. Moreover, early induction of menopause in young women is associated with increased risk of osteoporosis and cardiovascular disease in later years.

It is interesting to note that the available evidence does not establish the relative roles of chemotherapy (the most commonly employed systemic adjuvant therapy for premenopausal breast cancer) and ovarian ablation. It has been suggested that chemotherapy may exert its beneficial effects merely by inducing ovarian ablation. However, there is also evidence to suggest that the beneficial effects of chemotherapy are seen even in the presence of continued ovarian function.

If this patient had an oestrogen receptor positive tumour, and was less than 5 years from her expected menopause, oophorectomy at the time of surgery would be reasonable, provided the issues of the management of menopausal symptoms have been considered and discussed with the patient. Outside these circumstances, ovarian ablation is not to be undertaken lightly.

3.8 Options to preserve fertility after treatment for breast cancer

A 34-year-old woman with early breast cancer has no children and wishes to retain the option of fertility after treatment of her malignancy. She is married, has been using an oral contraceptive for 10 years, and has never been pregnant. Treatment for her breast cancer will involve surgery, followed by local irradiation and adjuvant chemotherapy using drugs with the potential to induce premature ovarian failure. She may also be advised to have a bilateral oophorectomy.

What are her options for preservation of fertility?
Treatment of her breast cancer cannot be delayed to allow her to complete a pregnancy. This woman should be offered the chance to collect and store her oocytes to allow her the opportunity to conceive at a later date. It is also important that she should be aware, in making the decision to store genetic material, of her prognosis in relation to the stage of her disease. Pregnancy in a woman previously treated for breast cancer does not appear to have an adverse effect on the risk of breast cancer recurrence.

The options available to her include both proven and experimental choices under development. At present embryo cryostorage is the most proven and widely available. The first live birth after thawing and replacing a cryopreserved embryo was reported in 1981. Since then embryo freezing has become a routine part of IVF treatment programmes and many thousands of babies have been born as a result of this treatment. Embryos do not appear to be adversely affected by the length of cryostorage.

Creation of embryos requires the woman to complete a cycle of ovarian hyperstimulation followed by needle aspiration of ovarian follicles to obtain mature oocytes for *in vitro* fertilization. Embryos are usually cryostored after 1 or 2 days *in vitro* culture. The whole process takes approximately 2 weeks and must be done in accord with the time of the woman's menstrual cycle. This means it may take at least 1 month from the time of first planning to completion of the treatment. This may cause unacceptable delays in commencing cancer treatment. Creation and storage of embryos may not be appropriate for the single woman. It also creates significant moral and ethical problems relating to the long-term storage and eventual disposal of embryos for many women and their partners.

Cryostorage of mature oocytes collected after *in vivo* maturation avoid these problems. Immature or primary oocytes (which are present in large numbers in the ovarian cortex of a young woman) cannot be fertilized until they have reached metaphase II of meiosis. This occurs *in vivo* under the influence of gonadotrophins. In the follicular phase of a natural menstrual cycle, a single oocyte reaches maturity before ovulation. In order to collect several such oocytes simultaneously, exogenous gonadotrophins are used as part of assisted reproduction treatment cycles.

The major problem associated with collection and storage of mature oocytes is their potential to sustain damage during the process of cryo-preservation. Post-thaw survival and *in vitro* fertilization rates for these cells is low and to date fewer than 20 live births world-wide have been recorded. Cryopreservation appears to harden the zona pellucida, decreasing the penetration of spermatozoa, and inhibiting embryonic hatching. This process may also damage the cell spindle with the risk of chromosomal loss and aneuploidy at the first maturation division.

Immature oocytes within primordial follicles are smaller than metaphase II oocytes. They are also less differentiated, possess fewer organelles, and lack a zona pellucida and cortical granules. Because they are arrested in prophase they carry a lower risk of cytogenetic damage during cryostorage. They may be stored frozen, either after enzymatic recovery or in thin slices of ovarian tissue. However, immature oocytes require culture before becoming capable of fertilization and to date a proven, reliable *in vitro* culture system is not available.

There have been a number of successful animal experiments involving implantation of ovarian slices or autotransplantation of larger pieces of ovarian tissue. A return of normal ovarian function and pregnancies have been reported. Based on these results, many specialist fertility treatment centres have begun to freeze ovarian tissue from selected patients prior to chemotherapy or radiotherapy. Collection of ovarian tissue requires a laparoscopy which may be done at short notice without prior hormonal treatment.

At present, patients should be made aware of the possibility of cryo-storage of oocytes or ovarian tissue. However, they also need to be informed that this is still at the developmental stage and so far no human pregnancies have resulted from such measures.

3.9 Local recurrence after treatment for breast cancer

A 46-year-old woman underwent a modified radical mastectomy and axillary clearance for breast carcinoma some 4 years ago. Neither postoperative radio-therapy nor adjuvant systemic therapy were prescribed. On routine follow-up assessment two small (2–3 mm) nodules near the chest wall scar are detected. Fine needle aspiration confirms adenocarcinoma cells. The remainder of the physical examination proves normal. Chest radiograph, bone scan, and liver ultrasound are normal.

What is her prognosis and would this have been different if she had initially been treated by conservative surgery and breast irradiation?
Local recurrence is defined as tumour reappearing in ipsilateral breast, chest wall, or overlying skin after conservative surgery or mastectomy. Local recurrence after mastectomy is more often associated with metastatic disease on full staging than is local recurrence after conservation. Staging investigations should include chest CT, because chest wall or nodal recur-rence after mastectomy is characteristically associated with unsuspected disease in the internal mammary lymph nodes. Multiple involved nodes are most commonly seen under or near the second or third intercostal space.

Most patients with isolated local recurrence after mastectomy eventually develop distant metastases. The disease-free interval appears to be the most reliable predictor of subsequent survival. By contrast, local recurrence after breast conservation is generally regarded as having a better prognosis. A number of series report long-term disease-free survival after 'salvage' mastectomy in about 30 to 50 per cent of patients.

What are the options for treatment and, if the recurrence is apparently local only, would you recommend adjuvant systemic therapy at this point?
Radiotherapy would be appropriate in this case if no other disease is detected beyond the chest wall. The role of systemic 'adjuvant' therapy after radical irradiation of chest wall (plus or minus regional nodes) is not established. Although a number of centres have reported their experience

(small uncontrolled series) of 'adjuvant' systemic therapy, there is only one randomized trial addressing this issue. In that study, tamoxifen therapy after isolated locoregional relapse significantly increased 5-year disease-free survival rates from 36 per cent to 59 per cent (compared to observation alone).

Should more distant disease be detected, the relative benefits of chest wall irradiation versus systemic therapy should be considered.

If she had been treated by breast conservation, is it possible to tell whether reappearance of tumour represents recurrent disease or a new primary?
The short answer is USUALLY NOT!

Tumour appearing at or near a 'lumpectomy' site might be considered more likely to be recurrence than a new primary. Changes in histological appearance are of limited value, since changes in tumour grade may reflect the effects of prior radiation or chemotherapy.

Although only available in research laboratories, molecular technology can be used to determine the clonal origin of multiple tumours in female patients. Since tumours are monoclonal in origin, and since any given body cell in a female patient will have only one active X chromosome, a tumour may contain either an active paternally derived X chromosome or an active maternally derived X chromosome. If DNA from the original primary and the apparent recurrence are compared, and different (i.e. maternal versus paternal) X chromosomes are activated in the two tumours, then they must be separate primary tumours. However, if both tumours carry the same active X chromosome, two interpretations are possible. Either the 'recurrent' tumour is indeed a recurrence of the first, or the two tumours could have arisen independently, and by chance activated the same X chromosome. These latter two events are impossible to separate.

3.10 Spinal cord compression

You are following a 45-year-old woman with metastatic breast cancer involving the bones and liver. She has been well and symptom-free for 12 months on tamoxifen. At the end of the consultation, she mentions a vague hesitancy on commencing micturition, which she has assumed to be of no major consequence.

What thoughts should run through your mind?
In patients with malignancy, the astute clinician always carries a high index of suspicion for spinal cord compression. Symptoms are often vague in the early stages and easily missed. Check for mild disturbance of bowel and bladder function, back pain (especially radicular pain), and symptoms of gait disturbance. Patients with advanced cancer often have multiple aches and pains, and may not recognize the potential significance of these symp-

toms. Interestingly, patients with advanced neurological deficit from malignant cord compression often exhibit surprising indifference to their deficit. Cord compression is particularly common in advance breast and lung cancer. It is relatively uncommon in prostate cancer, despite often extensive bone metastases.

Focused clinical examination of the lower limb neurology and assessment of sensory deficit at a dermatomal level are necessary.

How would you investigate these symptoms?
Urgent MRI of the entire spinal column, and probably the cranium as well, is required. MRI is the preferred technique, where available, as it can assess the entire length of the spinal cord and associated bony structures, as well as lesions that do not cause thecal sac compression or bony distortion. It is appropriate to scan the cranium as well, as multiple cerebral metastases may also be present.

Where MRI is not readily available, myelography followed by CT scanning through areas of abnormality is the investigation of choice. Myelography carries some risk of sudden neurological deterioration after lumbar puncture, but does allow the collection of cerebrospinal fluid for biochemical and cytological analysis.

Consider commencing the patient on dexamethasone whilst awaiting the results of investigations.

MRI scan reveals an epidural mass centred on the body of T6, extending into both pedicles and compromising 50 per cent of the spinal canal diameter.

How should this woman be treated?
Intervention is required to preserve neurological function. For most solid tumours, radiotherapy and surgery offer equal efficacy. Surgery, however, is preferred if there is doubt about a tissue diagnosis, or if there is a neurological deficit due to compression by bone rather than tumour (e.g. compression fracture with a retro-pulsed fragment). Surgery should also be considered if there is progression despite radiotherapy. Radiotherapy is preferred if the tumour type is highly radiosensitive, for example lymphoma or small cell lung cancer.

The prognosis of the cord compression relates most closely to the degree of deficit before commencing therapy, emphasizing the need for high levels of clinical suspicion and early diagnosis.

3.11 Major depression in a patient with breast cancer

A 46-year-old woman presents complaining that she feels chronically anxious and depressed. She has been treated for early breast cancer 6 months ago. She is worried that the cancer will return and cannot get this thought out of her mind.

How can you best help her?
All cancer patients will be depressed and anxious at some time or another. Clinicians must not only support their patients through crises, but also try to determine when their distress reaches a level that merits specific treatment.

There are two types of depression. The first is the sort of depression that anyone will feel when something bad happens. This **reactive depression** is a normal reaction to being told that one has cancer. It requires no more intervention than simple support and encouragement and tends to resolve as time passes. The second sort of depression, known as **major depression**, is not a normal reaction. It is a clinical syndrome that has a biological basis. Major depression demands specific treatment. It may arise from, and complicate, reactive depression, but those with major depression tend to feel worse as time goes by, rather than better. Eventually the patient with major depression may feel that they have entered a dark pit which permits no exit other than suicide.

Studies suggest that major depression frequently occurs in oncology patients (as high as 30 per cent in some series), but that it is frequently overlooked. The clinician should be alert to the possibility that their sad or anxious patients might have a major depression and avoid explaining away their symptoms with the oft heard 'anyone would be depressed in their situation'.

Diagnosing major depression in the patient with cancer is made difficult by considerable overlap of symptoms of depression and of cancer. Lethargy, sleep disturbance, appetite disturbance, and weight loss may all occur with both. There are some features, though, that are more suggestive of a major depression and should raise clinical suspicion when present. Though many cancer patients will frequently feel depressed, feeling sad all, or almost all, of the time suggests a major depression. Similarly clinically depressed patients may report that nothing can cheer them up and that they often feel they are at their worst in the morning. Major depression typically causes a particular type of sleep disturbance. Classically patients will wake at 3.00am or 4.00am and, unable to return to sleep, will lie in bed and darkly ruminate about their future. Any patient in whom a mood disturbance is suspected must be asked specifically if they have considered suicide and what plans they have made. Remember too that delirium may resemble depression and that depression may be a side-effect of numerous medications.

The management of major depression starts with reassuring the patient and educating them about the illness that has complicated their cancer. The patient should know that major depression is common and that it will almost certainly improve with treatment. Reassure them that having major depression in no way implies that they are inadequate. Rather, inform them that they have a disease where the chemicals in their brains controlling their moods have become unbalanced and it is this imbalance that is making them abnormally depressed.

The comprehensive management of a major depression involves far more than just the simple dispensing of antidepressants. Psychological interventions such as supportive listening and cognitive behavioural strategies are very important. For most patients, though, the back bone of management will be antidepressant medication. Generally the newer antidepressants, such as selective serotonin reuptake inhibitors, are to be preferred over older tricyclic antidepressants because of their more favourable side-effect profiles. Warn the patient that the drug will not have any effect for a week or two.

Generally patients will respond well within 3 to 4 weeks, and should then be continued on the drug at the same dose for around 6 to 9 months. Patients who do not respond should be referred to a consultation-liaison psychiatrist

3.12 Managing cancer pain

A 56-year-old woman with metastatic breast cancer complains of a localized posterior neck pain that is aggravated by turning her head. It has been present for several weeks and is getting worse. She is taking ten codeine/paracetamol compound analgesic tablets per day with little benefit. The patient has been treated for metastatic breast cancer for 5 years, and has been treated with several endocrine manipulations and chemotherapy. She recently underwent a right hip replacement because of metastatic disease in her femur at risk of pathological fracture.

What can you do to improve her pain control?
Bone metastases to the cervical spine are almost certainly the cause of the pain in this woman's case, and the first step in her management is to take a thorough pain history (site, intensity, and other characteristics of the pain, treatment history), perform a focused physical examination (including a careful neurological examination in this case), and order appropriate investigations (plain radiograph, bone scan, and possibly MRI) to confirm the clinical suspicion.

A strong opioid such as morphine is needed because a weak opioid (codeine) has been ineffective. Codeine 60 mg by mouth is approximately equivalent to 10 mg oral morphine, so she should be commenced on morphine mixture (immediate release solution) 10 mg, 4-hourly. Addition of adjuvant analgesics, such as paracetamol or a non-steroidal anti-inflammatory, can be opioid sparing and improve the quality of analgesia for bone pain, so paracetamol 1 gm four times a day and naproxen 1 gm/day should be added. The dose of morphine mixture may need to be titrated up to achieve an effective dose, but most patients need no more than 200 mg/day. Once a stable effective dose is achieved, a sustained release preparation should be used to improve compliance. Laxatives (e.g. coloxyl and senna twice a day) should be administered prophylactically, to prevent opioid-induced constipation.

Physical therapy may also have a role (e.g. soft collar, hot packs). Antitumour treatment is an important part of the treatment of cancer pain such as this, and a radiation oncology consultation should be arranged.

Strong opioid analgesics remain the mainstay of the pharmacological management of moderate to severe cancer pain. Morphine is now commercially available in several forms, including immediate release solutions and tablets, sustained release tablets and capsules, and ampoules for injection. Familiarity with the specific use of each formulation is needed, and a full account is beyond the scope of this commentary. Suggested guidelines for the correct use of morphine for chronic cancer pain are as follows:

- give by mouth, if possible;
- give on a time-contingent, regularly-scheduled basis, not 'as required';
- start with immediate-release solution at a dose of 5 to 10 mg 4-hourly, titrate dose up in a stepwise fashion until the pain is relieved or intolerable side-effects occur;
- when an effective dose is reached, convert to a sustained-release preparation at the same total dose;
- use rescue doses (100 per cent of 4-hourly dose) for 'breakthrough pain';
- dosage may need to be adjusted up or down subsequently—dose reduction is usually required if a noxious stimulus is removed (e.g. radiotherapy for bone metastases or successful nerve block), or renal impairment leads to accumulation of active metabolites;
- provide prophylaxis of side-effects—laxatives are usually needed, antiemetics are needed infrequently;
- if parenteral administration is necessary, use the subcutaneous route— subcutaneous morphine is twice as potent as oral morphine;
- if changing to a different opioid, the relative potency ratio of each needs to be considered;
- patient and carer fears about morphine addiction need to be discussed and allayed.

Side-effects are common when opioid therapy is being initiated, but remain troublesome in only a minority of patients. Drowsiness and dizziness usually resolve after a few days. Nausea only affects a minority of patients and usually resolves after a few days. Prophylactic laxatives to prevent opioid-induced constipation are an essential part of initiating management with opioids. Substitution of another strong opioid (such as oxycodone, methadone, or fentanyl) may be tried if morphine is ineffective or poorly tolerated, although pethidine should not be used for chronic cancer pain.

Pain in patients with cancer may not just be due to the disease but can be a side-effect of treatment (e.g. post-thoracotomy pain syndrome), or unrelated to the cancer (e.g. back pain due to an old work injury or osteoporosis). It is also important to remember that cancer pain is not a homogeneous entity and patients often experience multiple pains simultaneously. Each one has to be identified and individually assessed. Classifying cancer pain into its common syndromes (e.g. base of skull syndromes, vertebral syndromes, liver capsule pain, retroperitoneal pain, plexopathy pain) is helpful, and can hasten the initiation of appropriate treatment modalities.

A psychosocial evaluation of the patient and carer is also needed, to identify issues which might modify pain responses. Fears of tolerance and addiction to pain killers, fear of progressive disease, and reluctance to bother the staff by complaining about pain all need to be identified and managed. Use of a tool such as a rating scale or brief pain questionnaire aids pain assessment and treatment, but these may not be possible to use with very sick, distressed, or elderly patients. While it is essential that the pain assessment be as comprehensive as possible, this should not delay the initiation of analgesic therapy. Treatment must be offered during pain assessment, even if some adjustment is needed once the assessment is completed.

On-going reassessment and adjustment of treatment is an important part of optimal pain management. Follow-up assessments are necessary to evaluate the durability of pain relief. Changes in pain patterns or new pain requires a new diagnostic work-up (e.g. onset of radicular pain to the occipital region, neck, or shoulder in this patient requires exclusion of epidural disease).

In 5 per cent of patients, cancer pain becomes refractory to standard treatment. Even neuroablation is ineffective. Many of these patients are individuals who are truly suffering and conceptualize their existential distress as physical pain. Ultimately, medicine can not have the answer to all the suffering of life and death. Our challenge is to understand the nature of such suffering and be empathetic to it. Suffering has been described as 'an awareness of the disintegration of self'. Our goal is to relieve the medical aspects of that sense of loss of personhood and not to contribute further to it.

The patient returns to the clinic a month later complaining of a paroxysmal burning pain that shoots up the back of the her head when she nods. She has taken several breakthrough doses of morphine, which have made her drowsy but have not reduced her pain.

What can you do to improve her pain control?
The patient now has a neuropathic pain, presumably due to progressive disease with compression of the C1–2 nerve roots by tumour. Neuropathic

pain is distinguished from nociceptive pain by its clinical characteristics which relate to differences in the pathophysiological mechanism. Nociceptive pain is due to a noxious stimulus from damaged somatic or visceral structures, and is transmitted via the nervous system. Neuropathic pain arises in damaged nervous tissue, and need not be associated with a noxious stimulus in the periphery.

Changes in the pattern of chronic cancer pain or the onset of new pain such as this requires a new diagnostic work-up (e.g. onset of radicular pain to the occipital region, neck, or shoulder in this patient requires exclusion of epidural disease). A thorough pain history (site, intensity, and other characteristics of the pain), a focused physical examination (including a careful neurological examination in this case) and appropriate investigations (plain radiograph, bone scan, possibly MRI) are needed. Although a C1–2 radiculopathy is most likely, cervical cord compression, postradiotherapy neuropathy, and bone metastases to the skull are differential diagnoses. Other diagnoses such as tension headache or migraine need to be considered, although the clinical presentation should clearly distinguish them.

If the investigations reveal an epidural deposit, meningeal disease, or a pathological fracture of a cervical vertebra, these abnormalities may become the target for therapy with antitumour treatments, especially if this is the only problem in an otherwise well patient. Frequently, however, this is not the case, either because no such specific problem can be identified or the disease is so far advanced that the burden and risks of intervention outweigh the potential benefits. In such cases, amelioration of the neuropathic pain becomes the primary goal of treatment.

Although neuropathic pain is said to be unresponsive to opioid analgesics, this is not entirely true. All patients with neuropathic pain should have a trial of these agents if they are not already doing so, not only because neuropathic pain may respond to opioids but also because patients with metastatic cancer rarely have isolated neuropathic pain syndromes (unlike patients with postherpetic neuralgia, diabetic neuropathy, or tic doloreux). For patients already on opioids, the dose should be increased until the pain is relieved or intolerable side-effects occur. For patients not responding to opioids, options include adjuvant analgesics and anaesthetic techniques.

Numerous agents in diverse drug classes have been recommended for treating neuropathic pain, though the science supporting their use is limited. Commonly used agents include tricyclic antidepressants (e.g. amitryptilline), anticonvulsant (e.g. sodium valproate, carbemazepine, gabapentin), and oral local anaesthetics (e.g. mexilitine, flecainide). Other agents that have occasionally been tried include corticosteroids and NMDA receptor antagonists (ketamine, dextromethorphan). Recent evidence suggests that methadone may have activity as an NMDA antagonist.

Although anecdotal evidence suggests that favourable responses may be obtained with these agents, the clinician must recognize that use of these drugs is limited by problems of adverse effects, comorbidities, drug interactions, and contributing to polypharmacy. This is particularly the case if agents from several classes are used concurrently.

In this patient's case, if the paroxysmal pain persisted after optimization of the morphine dose, an agent such as amitryptilline or valproate would be the first choice, depending on her other symptoms and comorbidities. These should be titrated up to full antidepressant/anticonvulsant doses if tolerated (i.e. 100 to 150 mg/day amitryptilline or 1500 to 2000 mg/day valproate). If this proves ineffective, flecainide (50 mg two times per day initially, increasing to 100 mg three times per day) could be tried, provided there is no history of ischaemic heart disease or evidence of myocardial dysfunction. Alternatively, a subcutaneous ketamine infusion (250 mg/day, increasing to 400 mg/day if tolerated) could be tried. Changing the morphine to methadone would also be reasonable.

If these drug manoeuvres proved ineffective, an anaesthetic technique (nerve block or spinal opioids) should be considered (see Cases 8.6 and 8.8).

References

3.1

Hoskins, K. F., Stopfer, J. E., Calzone, K. A., *et al.* (1995). Assessment and counseling for women with a family history of breast cancer. *Journal of the American Medical Association*, **273**, 577–585.

3.2

Breast Cancer Prevention Trial Protocol P1 (unpublished). Available in brief on the Internet at http://cancertrials.nci.nih.gov.

Early Breast Cancer Trialist's Collaborative Group (1998). Tamoxifen for early breast cancer: an overview of the randomised trials. *Lancet*, **351**, 1451–1467.

Powles, T., Eeles, R., Ashley, S. *et al.* (1998). Interim analysis of the incidence of breast cancer in the Royal Marsden Hospital tamoxifen randomised chemo-prevention trial. *Lancet*, **352**, 98–101.

Veronesi, U., Maisonneuve, P., Costa, A. *et al.* (1998). Prevention of breast cancer with tamoxifen: preliminary findings from the Italian randomised trial among hysterectomised women. *Lancet*, **352**, 93–97.

3.3

Boyages, J., Connolly, J.L., Schnitt, S.J., and Harris, J.R. (1977). Definition of an extensive intraductal component. Appendix 5 in Australian Cancer Network Breast Cancer Pathology Working Party. *The pathology reporting of breast cancer. A guide for pathologists, surgeons, and radiologists.* Australian Cancer Network, Sydney.

Holland, R., Connolly, J.L., Gelman, R., *et al.* (1990). The presence of an extensive intraductal component following a limited excision correlates with prominent residual disease in the remainder of the breast. *Journal of Clinical Oncology*, **8**, 113–118.

Schnitt, S.J., Connolly, J.L., Harris, J.R., *et al.* (1984). Pathologic predictors of early local recurrence in Stage I and II breast cancer treated by primary radiation therapy. *Cancer*, **53**, 1049–1057.

3.4

Kollmorgen, D.R., Varanasi, J.S., Edge, S.B. *et al.* (1998). Paget's disease of the breast: a 33 year experience. *Journal of the American College of Surgery*, **187**, 171–177.

Pierce, L.J., Haffty, B.G., Solin, L.J. *et al.* (1997). The conservative management of Paget's disease of the breast with radiotherapy. *Cancer*, **80**, 1065–1072.

Yim, J.H., Wick, M.R., Philpott, G.W. *et al.* (1997). Underlying pathology in mammary Paget's disease. *Annals of Surgery and Oncology*, **4**, 287–92.

3.5

Overgaard, M., Hansen, P., Overgaard, J. *et al.* (1997). Postoperative radiotherapy in high risk premenopausal women with breast cancer who receive adjuvant chemotherapy. *New England Journal of Medicine*, **337**, 949–955.

Ragaz, J., Jackson, S., Le, N. *et al.* (1997). Adjuvant radiotherapy and chemotherapy In node-positive premenopausal women with breast cancer. *New England Journal of Medicine*, **337**, 956–962.

Recht, A., Bartelink, H., Fourquet, A. *et al.* (1998). Postmastectomy radiotherapy: questions for the twenty-first century. *Journal of Clinical Oncology*, **16**, 2886–2889.

3.6

Early Breast Cancer Trialist's Collaborative Group (1998*a*). Polychemotherapy for early breast cancer: an overview of the randomised trials. *Lancet*, **352**, 930–942.

Early Breast Cancer Trialist's Collaborative Group (1998*b*). Tamoxifen for early breast cancer: an overview of the randomised trials. *Lancet*, **351**, 1451–1467.

Piccart, M.J., Biganzoli, L., and Roy, J.A. (1996). Adjuvant systemic therapy for breast cancer. *Current Opinions in Oncology*, **8**, 478–484.

3.7

Early Breast Cancer Trials Group (1996). Ovarian ablation in early breast cancer; overview of the randomised trial. *Lancet*, **348**, 1189–1196.

3.8

Kroman, N., Jensen, M.B., Melbye, M. *et al.* (1997). Should women be advised against pregnancy after breast-cancer treatment? *Lancet*, **350**, 319–322.

Oktay, K., Newton, H., Aubard, Y., *et al.* (1998). Cryopreservation of immature human oocytes and ovarian tissue: an emerging technology? *Fertilization and Sterilization*, **69**, 1–7.

3.9

Harris, J.R., Lippman, M.E., Morrow, M., and Hellman, S. (eds) (1996). *Diseases of the breast*. Lippincott-Raven: Philadelphia, New York.

3.10

Faul, C.M. and Flickinger, J.C. (1995). The use of radiation in the management of spinal metastases. *Journal of Neurological Oncology*, **23**, 149–161.

Schiff, D., Batchelor, T., and Wen, PY. (1998). Neurologic emergencies in cancer patients. *Neurological Clinics*, **16**, 449–483.

3.11

Fawzy, F.I., Fawzy, N.W., Arndt, L.A. *et al.* (1995). Critical review of psychosocial interventions in cancer care. *Archives of General Psychiatry*, **52**, 100–113.

Lishman, W.A. (1998). *Organic Psychiatry. The psychological consequences of cerebral disorder*. Blackwell Science: London.

Rodin, G., Craven, J., and Littlefield, C. (1991). *Depression in the medically ill: an integrated clinical approach*. Bmnner/Mazel: New York.

3.12

Foley, K.M. (1998). Pain assessment and cancer pain syndromes. In *Oxford textbook of palliative medicine* (ed. Doyle, D., Hanks, G.W., and Macdonald, N.) (2nd edn), pp. 310–31. Oxford University Press.

Levy, M. (1996). Pharmacological management of cancer pain. *New England Journal of Medicine*, **335**, 1124–1132.

Portenoy, R.K. (1992). Cancer pain: pathophysiology and syndromes. *Lancet*, **339**, 1026–1031.

Portenoy, R.K. (1993). Adjuvant analgesics in pain management. In *Oxford textbook of palliative medicine* (ed. Doyle, D., Hanks, G.W., and Macdonald, N.) (2nd edn), pp. 187–203. Oxford University Press.

Zancy, J.P. (1993). A review of the effects of opioids on psychomotor and cognitive functioning in humans. *Experimental and Clinical Psychopharmacology*, **3**, 432–466.

4.1 Melanoma

A 43-year-old woman had a wide excision, skin graft, and prophylactic inguinal lymph node dissection as primary treatment of a melanoma on the left calf 3 years ago. The tumour was Clarke Level IV and 2.2 mm in depth with 1/17 inguinal lymph nodes positive. On routine follow-up, you detect a new flesh-coloured nodule above the left knee. On questioning, she admits to 2 months of intermittent cramping lower abdominal pain.

What is the purpose of follow-up in patients following resection of primary melanoma?
The purpose of follow-up is:

(1) the detection and treatment of salvageable locoregional recurrence, such as in transit metastasis or lymph node recurrence;
(2) the detection of second primary melanomas, and other non-melanoma skin cancers, for both of which there is an increased risk in patients who have had one primary melanoma.

The frequency and duration of follow-up is determined by the thickness of the primary melanoma, which also determines prognosis (Table 4.1).

Table 4.1 Relationship between thickness of the primary tumour and prognosis

Pathological stage	10-year survival (%)
pTis—Melanoma *in situ*	100
pTI—Melanoma ≤0.75 mm thick	97.9
pT2—Melanoma >0.75–1.5 mm thick	90.7
pT3a— Melanoma >1.5–3.0 mm thick	75.4
pT3b—pT4—Melanoma >3.0 mm thick	55.0

What influence did the prophylactic lymph node dissection have on her prospects of survival?
Probably none.

There are now good data from large, randomized, controlled clinical trials to show that there is no survival benefit from prophylactic lymph node dissection following excision of primary limb melanomas. This contrasts with data from earlier, historically controlled trials that did suggest a benefit.

Lymph node dissection is still recommended management of clinically involved lymph nodes. Even when two to three lymph nodes are involved, 10-year survival rates of up to 30 per cent are reported. The technique of sentinel node biopsy (SNB) is currently being used to detect subclinical lymph node involvement. Patients are being randomized to either SNB± lymph node dissection or observation to test the value of prophylactic dissection in this selected group. There are no good data on the efficacy of prophylactic irradiation of regional nodes.

Would her chances of relapse and survival have been increased by the use of adjuvant systemic therapy following her initial surgery?
Maybe!

A large variety of agents have been tested as adjuvant treatments following definitive surgical management of high-risk primary melanoma including cytotoxic drugs, BCG vaccinations, levamisole, and vaccines prepared from cultured melanoma cells. Whilst major advances are currently being made in vaccine design, the only form of adjuvant treatment to have shown a survival advantage in prospective, randomized, controlled trials is interferon-α-2b. In large doses (20 MU/m^2 per day intravenously for 1 month followed by 10 MU/m^2 three times per week subcutaneously for 48 weeks) interferon-α-2b produced a 12-month increment in median overall survival (p<0.02). Although expensive, interferon treatment compares favourably with other cancer interventions in cost effectiveness. Interferon therapy is toxic, with approximately one-half of the interferon treated patients requiring major dose reductions. However, 'quality-of-life-adjusted time gained' outweighed the reduced quality of life associated with treatment toxicity and relapse. Further confirmation of this single study is awaited in the Intergroup 1690 study before standard adoption of this intensive and expensive adjuvant therapy. Meanwhile, wherever possible, eligible patients should be entered on randomized clinical trials of adjuvant therapy.

What is the likely diagnosis of the new nodule and how should it be managed?
The new nodule is likely to be a melanoma metastasis. Melanoma cells may settle 'in transit' along the lymphatic draining vessels between the primary tumour and the regional lymph nodes. From such seeding a local growth may occur at a later date. These may or may not be pigmented, whether or not the primary tumour was melanotic. A second primary, amelanotic melanoma is a differential diagnosis.

Management of an isolated 'in-transit' metastasis is wide excision without skin graft. Multiple 'in transit' metastases are best managed by isolated limb perfusion (i.e. perfusion of the limb with high concentrations of cytotoxics in combination with hyperthermia) which offers complete remission in over 70 per cent of patients. A long-term, disease-free state in the limb is achieved, with or without further treatment, in over 60 per cent of those sustaining an initial complete remission. The surgical access for this procedure is however highly invasive and time consuming. A similar technique using percutaneously placed catheters has recently been developed. While the hyperthermia induced is not as marked, the morbidity is considerably less. These techniques can be repeated.

How would you investigate the abdominal pain?
This should be investigated by high resolution abdominal CT plus or minus small bowel series. Laparotomy may be indicated in certain circumstances.

Melanoma is associated with a wide variety of metastatic patterns, and every organ has been known to be affected, including testis, breast, muscle, and retina. Knowledge of some of the most characteristic of these metastatic patterns assists in the interpretation and investigation of symptoms in following-up patients following treatment of high-risk primary melanoma. Particularly common sites of involvement are the subcutis, lymph nodes, lung, liver, and brain. One site favoured by melanoma and yet uncommonly by other solid tumours is the intestinal mucosa. Mucosal metastases present with bleeding or obstruction. Obstructive symptoms are often subacute, with episodic cramping abdominal pain, nausea, vomiting, and sometimes constipation. Mucosal metastases can be very difficult to image, although small bowel series and high resolution CT scanning are complementary. In certain cases, where symptoms are progressive and disabling and where clinical suspicion is high, laparoscopy and/or laparotomy may be indicated if the above investigations have proved negative, with a view to resection of bowel segment(s) containing mucosal metastases. Recovery from small intestinal procedures is usually quite rapid.

Resection of the nodule confirms an 'in transit' metastasis. CT scanning of the abdomen and small bowel series are both negative and the abdominal pain settles spontaneously. Three months later, a chest radiograph, performed during an incidental upper respiratory tract infection, reveals an isolated 2.5 cm nodule in the left upper lobe of the lung, which is confirmed on chest CT.

How would you manage the pulmonary metastasis?
The presence of other metastases should be excluded. Obtain a careful clinical history, paying special attention to any history of weight loss, anorexia, lethargy, or headache. Perform a careful physical examination, including wide palpation for subcutaneous metastases (running the palms of the hands over the entire skin surface), examination of the oropharynx, digital examination of the rectum, and neurological examination, including fundoscopy. Perform full blood count, liver function tests, serum lactate dehydrogenase, CT of chest, head, abdomen, and pelvis. Where available, gallium scanning and positron emission tomographic (PET) scanning provide very sensitive tools for the detection of metastatic disease.

Confirmation of isolated pulmonary metastasis is an indication for surgical resection. Surgical resection of an isolated metastasis may provide good palliation and, in a small proportion of cases, long-term survival. Resection should be considered for isolated pulmonary, cerebral, small intestinal, regional node, and some intraperitoneal recurrences.

Should 'adjuvant' systemic treatment be administered after resection of the pulmonary metastasis?

There is no evidence that the administration of systemic chemotherapy or immunotherapy after resection of isolated visceral metastases prolongs relapse free or overall survival, although this is the subject of a number of randomized, controlled clinical trials. In order to support these trials, and because the status of management of advanced melanoma is rapidly changing, the Australian Cancer Network Guidelines for the Management of Cutaneous Melanoma recommend that all such patients be referred for consultation in a multidisciplinary melanoma treatment centre. Whole brain radiotherapy is often given following resection of isolated cerebral metastases, on Level IV evidence only.

PET scanning prior to the planned pulmonary resection reveals multiple small pulmonary metastases and scattered retroperitoneal lymph node involvement.

Should the patient be offered systemic treatment?
Probably not.

There is no evidence that any form of systemic therapy prolongs overall survival for patients with disseminated metastatic melanoma. It is therefore advisable not to screen for other asymptomatic metastatic disease, and to reserve systemic therapy for patients who are either symptomatic, show early signs of weight loss, or who display rapid tumour progression. Regrettably, in a disease in which a principle objective is palliation, there are few reports of the effect of chemotherapy on quality of life. Such studies are now in progress.

The patient states that she cannot accept an observation policy and that she would like a referral to an oncologist who will 'do something.'

How may patients be persuaded that observation may be in their best interests whilst they remain asymptomatic?

The following arguments may be of benefit in persuading a patient that the relative risks and benefits of chemotherapy may, on balance, favour observation in the early asymptomatic stages of the disease:

- Chemotherapy may 'impair' the natural immune response. There is a well-documented spontaneous remission rate in melanoma of approximately 0.5 per cent. Sites associated with a better prognosis include subcutis, skin, lung, and lymph nodes.

- Chemotherapy is like 'money in the bank' and will be equally effective at any stage of the disease.
- Advise sensible simple dietary attention, perhaps with the aid of a nutritionist colleague: bolster antioxidant intake.
- Advise gentle exercise, avoiding fatigue.
- Advise relaxation therapy or massage.

After 3 months of remaining quite well, the patient develops dyspnoea on exertion and the chest radiograph shows progression in the multiple pulmonary nodules.

What systemic therapy should she be offered and what are the expected outcomes of treatment?
Single agent chemotherapy with dacarbazine (DTIC) should be offered.

Metastatic melanoma is relatively resistant to treatment with cytotoxic drugs. Partial responses to single agents occur in less than 25 per cent of treated patients, and complete responses in less than 5 per cent. The single agent with the highest reproducible response rate is DTIC with responses of 15 to 20 per cent. These responses are usually short lived ($<$ 6 months). The usual schedule is 750 mg/m^2 intravenous bolus third weekly. Temozolamide is a new DTIC analogue which is administered orally and which may have equivalent efficacy. Other single agents with some activity against melanoma (15 to 20 per cent response rate) are the nitrosoureas (BCNU, CCNU, and fotemustine), the vinca alkaloids (vincristine, vinblastine, and vindesine), cisplatin, and the taxanes (taxol and taxotere). Despite many initial reports of higher response rates in Phase II studies of a variety of combinations, there is currently no randomized, controlled trial evidence to support the superiority of any combination regimen over single agent DTIC alone. Recent claims for high responses to biochemotherapy regimens utilizing cisplatin, vinblastine, and dacarbazine (CVD regimen) followed by rIFN-α and rIL-2 (response rate of 60 per cent and a complete response rate of 20 per cent) await the results of controlled trials comparing this regimen to DTIC alone before it can be recommended as standard therapy. Such trials will require careful comparison of quality of life indices, as the toxicity of the biochemotherapy regimen is high and includes severe myelosuppression, infections, IL-2 induced constitutional toxicity, and hypotension, such that 15 per cent of patients require intensive care support. Such toxicity is, of course, unacceptable when the principal objective of treatment is palliation and improvement in quality of life.

The current, first-line recommendation, then, for patients with symptomatic metastatic disease, outside of clinical trials, is single agent DTIC, which is simple, ambulatory, and associated with minimal toxicity when administered with modern antiemetics. Alopecia does not occur with DTIC therapy.

Wherever possible, patients with metastatic melanoma should be referred to melanoma centres for inclusion in clinical trials.

References

Atkins, M.B. (1997). The treatment of metastatic melanoma with chemotherapy and biologics. *Current Opinions in Oncology*, **9**, 205–13.

Australian Cancer Network (1997). *Guidelines for the management of cutaneous melanoma*. Stone Press: Epping.

Balch, C.M. *et al.* (1998). *Cutaneous melanoma* (3rd edn). Quality Medical Publishing Company: St Louis, M.O.

Cole, B.F., Gelber, R.D., Kirkwood, J.M. *et al.* (1996). Quality-of-life-adjusted survival analysis of interferon alfa-2b adjuvant treatment of high-risk resected cutaneous melanoma: an Eastern Cooperative Oncology Group study. *Journal of Clinical Oncology*, **14**, 2666–2673.

Kirkwood, J. M., Strawderman, M.H., Ernstoff, M.S. *et al.* (1996). Interferon alfa-2b adjuvant therapy of high-risk resected cutaneous melanoma: the Eastern Cooperative Oncology Group Trial EST 1684 [see comments]. *Journal of Clinical Oncology*, **14**, 7–17.

Legha, S.S., Ring, S., Bedikian, A. *et al.* (1996). Treatment of metastatic melanoma with combined chemotherapy containing cisplatin, vinblastine and dacarbazine (CVD) and biotherapy using interleukin-2 and interferon-alpha. *Annals of Oncology*, 7, 827–835.

Rosenberg, S.A., Yang, J.C., Schwartzentruber, D.J. *et al.* (1998). Immunologic and therapeutic evaluation of a synthetic peptide vaccine for the treatment of patients with metastatic melanoma. *Nature Medicine*, **4**, 321–327.

Thompson, J.F., Hunt, J.A., Shannon, K.F. *et al.* (1997). Frequency and duration of remission after isolated limb perfusion for melanoma. *Archives of Surgery*, **132**, 903–907.

Haematological oncology

5.1 A young woman with early-stage Hodgkin's disease

A 32-year-old woman has noticed a lump in her neck for 3 weeks. She is otherwise well, with no previous illnesses. She reports no night sweats, fevers, or weight loss. On examination, you detect a 5-cm, left-sided, supraclavicular mass together with a 2.5-cm, left-sided, cervical node. There were no other significant clinical findings. A chest radiograph reveals a widened upper mediastinum, but to less than one-third (0.35) of the chest diameter. A blood count and film is normal, but her erythrocyte sedimentation rate (ESR) is raised at 60 mm/h. Serum biochemistry and liver function tests are normal. A thoracic CT scan demonstrates mediastinal lympha- denopathy measuring 6 cm in diameter, together with a 2-cm subcarinal lymph node. An abdominal CT scan is entirely normal. Cervical lymph node biopsy confirms nodular sclerosing Hodgkin's disease. On gallium scan there is increased tracer uptake on the left side of the neck, and in the mediastinum. There was no gallium avidity seen elsewhere. A bone marrow aspirate and trephine are normal.

Has this patient been staged sufficiently?
Appropriate staging investigations include chest radiograph and CT scan of chest, abdomen, and pelvis, and high-dose gallium scans. Previously, staging laparotomy and splenectomy were performed in an attempt to detect micro- scopic disease that would elevate apparent stage II patients to stage III, who were considered best treated with chemotherapy rather than radiotherapy. However, pathological staging is no longer performed because:

- treatment has to be delayed for nearly 3 weeks;
- the morbidity associated with laparotomy and splenectomy is not trivial;
- splenectomy increases the risk of life-threatening infection with encapsu- lated organisms;
- patients who relapse after radiotherapy can be effectively treated with chemotherapy such that their overall survival is not compromised.

The Ann Arbor staging classification has been the basis for treatment decisions in Hodgkin's disease for more than 20 years. It was originally de- signed to distinguish patients who could be adequately treated with extended field radiotherapy from those requiring systemic chemotherapy. The patient described here has stage IIA Hodgkin's disease by this classification.

How would you treat this patient?

The management of early-stage Hodgkin's disease is driven by the need to balance treatment toxicity, effectiveness, and long-term complications. Treatment decisions are based primarily upon disease subtype and accurate staging of extent. Conventional treatment of early-stage disease (I, II) consists of subtotal nodal irradiation (STNI), that is a supradiaphragmatic component (shaped like a polo neck sweater with short sleeves) followed by an infradiaphragmatic port (including the para-aortic lymph node area from T12 to L4, and the spleen). This results in long-term disease-free survival in up to 75 per cent of patients. Some experts argue that irradiation for Hodgkin's disease is a subspecialty, tertiary referral area of radiation oncology and that patients should be treated in specialist centres to achieve optimal results.

Although most patients with early-stage disease are cured with optimal radiation therapy, there is still a significant risk of relapse (up to 25 per cent), and even higher in the unfavourable prognostic group. Nevertheless, overall survival remains high (90 per cent) because of the effectiveness of salvage chemotherapy following relapses after radiotherapy.

Should this patient receive chemotherapy?

Yes!

Adding chemotherapy can reduce the risk of relapse after irradiation. For most patients, however, this represents over-treatment and increases the risk of long-term sequelae. Hence, the major controversy in treatment of Hodgkin's disease revolves around selection of patients with early-stage disease who are at higher than average risk of relapse and who might benefit from additional limited chemotherapy to prevent relapse and allow limited radiotherapy to prevent some of the long-term sequelae.

An EORTC (European Organization for Research and Treatment of Cancer) Lymphoma Cooperative Group analysis of trials in early-stage Hodgkin's disease, delineated three subsets with a very favourable, favourable, and an unfavourable prognosis (Table 5.1). Patients belonging to the very favourable and favourable subgroups treated with mantle field irradiation and STNI, respectively, can be expected to have a failure free

Table 5.1 EORTC prognostic groups in early stage Hodgkin's disease

Group	Prognostic features
Very favourable	Clinical Stage I *and* age < 40 years *and* Stage A and ESR < 50 *and* female *and* mediastinal:thoracic diameter ratio < 0.35
Favourable	All other patients not included in very favourable or unfavourable
Unfavourable	Age $\geqslant 50$ *or* stage A + ESR $\geqslant 50$ *or* stage B + ESR > 30 *or* clinical stage II with $\geqslant 4$ sites of disease *or* mediastinal:thoracic diameter ratio > 0.35

survival of at least 80 per cent and an overall survival of about 90 per cent at 6 years.

The patient described here has *unfavourable* stage IIA Hodgkin's disease, because she has four sites of involvement, a raised ESR (>50 mm/h), although the mediastinal lymph node mass measures less than 0.35 of the chest diameter. According to the EORTC criteria above, this would place her in the unfavourable prognostic group.

ABVD chemotherapy (*a*driamycin, *b*leomycin, *v*inblastine, and *d*acarbazine) appears to carry little risk of either secondary acute leukaemia or sterility, and has now gained widespread acceptance as standard chemotherapy for Hodgkin's disease. Other combinations of chemotherapy are being investigated in attempts to improve efficacy and/or reduce adverse effects. For example the MOPP/ABV (*m*ustine, *o*ncovin/vincristine, *pro*carbazine, and *p*rednisone) hybrid regimen combines multiple active agents, but with reduced doses of procarbazine and mustine compared to standard MOPP. However, demonstration of the superiority or otherwise of such regimens awaits mature results from current trials.

Where possible this patient should be treated on a clinical trial. If this is not practical, this patient would be best treated initially with chemotherapy (e.g. ABVD or MOPP/ABV) for a total of four courses, following which she should be restaged. If she is in partial remission, an additional two courses should be given followed by involved field radiotherapy to 30 (or 36) Gy. If she is in complete remission, then commencement of involved field radiotherapy can be undertaken after the initial four courses of chemotherapy.

Other current trials in unfavourable early-stage disease (e.g. German Hodgkin's Study Group HD8 and HD9 trials; EORTC H8 and H9 trials) are examining whether less than six courses of chemotherapy are required to achieve a complete remission if combined with involved field radiotherapy of 20 to 36 Gy. Alternative approaches in the unfavourable prognostic group include reducing the number of chemotherapy cycles (two to four) to reduce toxicity and to combine this with STNI to prevent relapses in initially uninvolved nodal areas (summarized in reference 4). Of course any reduction in relapse rate must be weighed against the induction of more secondary tumours, which can result from using larger radiotherapy fields. Only with data provided from results of the studies outlined above, will the long-term benefits and relative risks of each regimen be fully elucidated.

She is engaged to be married and is concerned about infertility from the chemotherapy. She is also concerned about her long-term prognosis. What would you tell her?

Although curves representing failure-free survival show a plateau after 5 to 7 years (which means that a late relapse of Hodgkin's disease is a very rare event) overall survival curves show that there is a constant decrease in the number of patients surviving. Even after 15 years from initial treatment, no plateau level can be demonstrated. This excess in mortality is mainly due to second malignancies and cardiac failure. Acute leukaemia is related solely to the given dose of MOPP therapy; the risk is not significantly increased for less than a total dose equivalent of one and a half cycles of MOPP.

The other long-term complication is an increased risk of solid tumours (e.g. breast, thyroid, lung, lymphoma, gastric, and colon carcinomas), for which the main risk factors are the extent of radiation therapy, and chemotherapy as sole treatment. Finally, cardiac failure has been shown to be dependent on radiation therapy rather than anthracycline toxicity.

Apart from these lethal treatment complications, there is a significant incidence of ovarian or testicular failure induced by MOPP chemotherapy in young patients. Men who receive more than three courses of MOPP are almost inevitably rendered sterile, while recovery to normal sperm counts occurs in most men who have had less than two courses of MOPP. As many as 70 per cent of women treated with six courses of MOPP become infertile, although younger patients (<26 years) are more likely to retain ovarian function. Since ABVD is associated with a low risk of infertility, it is the regimen of choice for young patients with Hodgkin's disease. (See Case 3.8 for a discussion of options for preservation of fertility).

5.2 Large cell non-Hodgkin's lymphoma

A 45-year-old male presents with a 4-week history of a right neck mass, recent weight loss of 5 kg, and drenching night sweats. On examination, there is a firm mass in the right supraclavicular fossa (SCF) measuring 2.5 cm with multiple smaller (1 cm) nodes elsewhere in both supraclavicular fossae and anterior cervical chains. There is no hepatosplenomegaly, nor epitrochlear, axillary, or inguinal lymphadenopathy. CT scans show mediastinal and hilar adenopathy with extensive retroperitoneal, para-aortic, and mesenteric nodes. Gallium-67 scan demonstrates gallium avidity in all these sites. Full blood count (FBC) results are haemoglobin (Hb) 127 g/l, white blood cells (WBC) 8.2×10^9/l, and platelets 330×10^9/l. The ESR is 120 mm/h with prominent rouleaux on blood film. Electrolytes are normal and lactate dehydrogenase (LDH) is elevated at 1600 U/l (NR 150 to 600 U/l). The bone marrow is mildly hypercellular with reactive changes but there was no evidence of malignancy. Biopsy of the right SCF lymph node was performed and reported as B-cell diffuse large cell lymphoma.

What is the preferred treatment and outlook for this man?
B-cell, diffuse large cell lymphoma is one of the more common forms of non-Hodgkin's lymphoma. In the 'Working Formulation' classification it was regarded as 'intermediate grade' but the more recent 'REAL' (*Revised European American Lymphoma* classification) combines 'centroblastic' and 'immunoblastic' categories, now considered to be essentially identical.

The disease usually requires aggressive therapy. The stage of disease (in this patient stage III B) is an important prognostic factor. The International non-Hodgkin's lymphoma Prognostic Factors Project identified four groups on the basis of age, stage, LDH, and performance status with predicted 5-year survival of 83 per cent, 69 per cent, 46 per cent, and 32 per cent respectively.

Combination chemotherapy with anthracycline containing regimens are standard therapy for diffuse large cell lymphoma. Multicentre clinical trials have demonstrated that the CHOP regimen (cyclophosphamide, hydroxy-daunorubicin, oncovin/vincristine, prednisone) results in complete clinical remission as effectively as more complex, toxic, and costly regimens such as MACOP-B (methotrexate, adriamycin, cyclophosphamide, oncarin, pre-clinisane, bleomycin) and ProMACE/CytaBOM (etoposide, adriamycin, cyclophosphamide, methotrexate, prednisone, cystesine, arabinoside, bleo-mycin, vincristine). CHOP remains standard therapy in most centres for diffuse large cell non-Hodgkin's lymphoma. Sites of bulky disease may require involved field radiotherapy to prevent relapse at these sites. Granulocyte colony stimulating factor (G-CSF) is commonly used prophy-lactically to minimize the degree and duration of neutropenia.

The patient is treated with six cycles of CHOP chemotherapy with G-CSF support, and achieves a complete remission on clinical grounds and on imaging. Follow-up at 6 months shows no sign of recurrence, but on review at 12 months, a new 6-cm retroperitoneal mass and para-aortic lymphadenopathy is seen with CT scanning. Gallium avidity is present in the abdomen and to a lesser extent in the mediastinum. A CT-guided fine needle aspiration biopsy of the retroperitoneal mass confirmed recurrence of large cell lymphoma.

How should he be treated now?

Relapse of disease is associated with a very poor prognosis and conventional chemotherapy alone does not achieve long-term disease-free survival. Salvage regimens such as DHAP (dexamethasone, high dose cytosine arabinoside, cisplatinum), ESHAP (etoposide, methylprednisolone, cytosine, cisplatinum) and others have been used but some 90 per cent of patients will ultimately relapse and die of their disease. In 1995, Philip et al. demonstrated improved survival for patients with chemotherapy-sensitive disease who underwent autologous bone marrow transplantation with event-free survival of 46 per cent in the transplant group compared to 12 per cent in the group receiving chemotherapy without transplantation.

Treatment is commenced using the DHAP regimen. Tumour chemosensitivity is confirmed with repeat CT scanning demonstrating good partial remission after two cycles of therapy. Peripheral blood stem cell (PBSC) harvesting is performed during recovery from cytopenia with G-CSF support. The patient remains alive in disease-free remission at 18 months following autografting.

How should he be followed up?
Follow-up intervals and investigations vary widely between clinicians and depend greatly on individual patient factors such as extent of disease, clinical symptoms and signs, and prognosis. Most physicians would review this patient at least three to four times annually for the first 1 to 2 years and then less frequently, usually with routine blood counts and biochemistry, including LDH. Diagnostic imaging with CT and perhaps gallium scanning would be utilized for some of these reviews depending on the site, stage, bulk, histology, imaging, and prognostic factors of the original disease and any new symptoms or signs. Fine needle aspiration biopsy may be useful to confirm disease recurrence and differentiate from other pathology and change in disease histology. (By contrast, it is often less useful at the time of original diagnosis as both cytology and lymph node architecture are required for accurate histological diagnosis.)

5.3 A 37-year-old with low grade lymphoma

A 37-year old man presents with a 6-week history of a progressively enlarging neck mass. He is otherwise well, with no previous illnesses. He describes night sweats over the last two nights only. On examination, there is a 6-cm mass low in the right cervical region, together with abnormal supraclavicular, cervical, axillary, and inguinal lymph nodes, each measuring up to 3 cm in diameter. His spleen is just palpable below the costal margin. A blood count, film, and routine biochemistry are normal, apart from a serum lactate dehydrogenase (LDH) of 960 U/l (NR 150 to 600 U/l). Chest radiograph is normal. A thoracic CT scan confirms the supraclavicular and axillary lymphadenopathy, together with small subcarinal and hilar lymph nodes (2 cm). An abdominal CT scan shows extensive para-aortic and mesenteric lymphadenopathy, as well as confirming the inguinal lymphadenopathy noted on examination. A gallium-67 scan shows diffuse, increased uptake in the neck, axillae, para-aortic, and inguinal regions. Bone marrow aspirate is unremarkable, but the marrow trephine shows several paratrabecular collections of lymphocytes which were positive for CD20 (L26) on immunoperoxidase staining. A cervical lymph node biopsy confirms follicular small cell non-Hodgkin's lymphoma. Immunophenotypic analysis of the lymph node using flow cytometry shows: CD19 = 85 per cent, CD20 = 88 per cent, CD5 negative, CD10 = 82 per cent, FMC-7 negative, kappa = 78 per cent. DNA analysis of both lymph node and bone marrow using enzymatic amplification by PCR was positive for the BCL-2 gene rearrangement.

How would you manage this case?
The patient has stage IV follicular low-grade non-Hodgkin's lymphoma which is clinically progressive in nature and from which he is symptomatic. A number of treatment options are available but need to be considered in the light of the natural history of the disease.

With a long median survival and a slow but continuous decrease in the survival curve, the low-grade lymphomas have previously been termed indolent or favourable. Despite high response rates with systemic therapy, these lymphomas are characterized by a pattern of continuous relapse and a median overall survival of 6 to 10 years. Hence, a policy of observation without systemic treatment until there is evidence of symptomatic progression is usually adopted. The exception to this rule is stage I disease which is sometimes curable with involved field radiotherapy.

Low grade lymphomas are exquisitely sensitive to a variety of therapies, including: alkylating agents (e.g. chlorambucil, cyclophosphamide) used as single agents; combination chemotherapy regimens cyclophosphamide, vincristine, and prednisone (CVP); or cyclophosphamide, hydroxydaunorubicin, oncovin/vincristine, and prednisone (CHOP); purine analogues; and local irradiation.

Purine analogues inhibit purine nucleotide metabolism resulting in accumulation of triphosphate metabolites which inhibit ribonucleotide reductase. They show response rates of 30 to 50 per cent in previously treated patients, and even higher in previously untreated patients. Included in this group of drugs are fludarabine, and 2-chlorodeoxyadenosine (2-CDA). The toxicity of purine analogues includes myelosuppression and infection with opportunistic organisms, including pneumocystis. All purine analogues lead to profound decreases in CD4 lymphocytes, often for prolonged periods (up to 23 to 40 months for recovery).

High-dose combination chemotherapy with autologous peripheral blood stem cell rescue (PBSC) has been used in patients with progressive or refractory disease, although it is too early to assess whether there is a significant survival benefit. Because of the systemic nature of low grade lymphoma, a large number of these patients will have bone marrow involvement, raising the possibility of reinfusing lymphoma cells during these procedures. Positive selection (CD34 cells) or negative selection (antibody purging) of harvested bone marrow or peripheral blood stem cells are approaches which have been used with variable success, but the risk of contaminating lymphoma cells is not eliminated. Allogeneic bone marrow transplantation offers the potential for cure, but because of its toxicity is limited to younger patients (i.e. < 55 years of age). Allogeneic transplantation may also allow development of a beneficial 'graft-versus-lymphoma' effect, as well as permitting delivery of very high doses of chemotherapy. Despite a high peritransplant mortality, preliminary studies are showing encouraging rates of disease-free survival.

Alpha-Interferon has been used either alone or in combination with chemotherapy, and has shown modest efficacy, with 30 to 50 per cent response rates as a single agent. At least five major, randomized studies of chemotherapy plus Alpha-interferon have demonstrated improvements in progression-free survival, but in only one was there a statistically significant improvement in overall survival. Even in this positive study, there remains the familiar pattern of continuous relapses, while the ostensible benefit in time to failure may be offset by the increased time on, and toxicity of, treatment.

Recently, a chimeric mouse/human anti-CD20 monoclonal antibody (Rituximab, Mabthera) has proved effective in relapsed low-grade NHL. Response rates of 50% were reported, with a median time to progression of 13 months. Rituximab combined with CHOP chemotherapy is currently being evaluated in relapsed low-grade NHL.

In this case, the patient opted for initial treatment with fludarabine. Tissue typing studies confirmed the availability of an HLA-matched sibling, such that on subsequent relapse allogenic bone marrow transplantation could be considered. Allogeneic transplantation may induce a 'graft-versus-lymphoma' effect which may help to induce prolonged disease-free survival in some patients with relapsed disease.

5.4 Two cases of chronic lymphocytic leukaemia (CLL)

Case one: A 62-year-old woman presents to her family doctor for a 'general check-up and a cholesterol test'. She was well and examination was entirely normal. A blood count was performed at the same time as the lipids and showed Hb 139 g/l, WBC 12.2×10^9/l, with lymphocytes 9.5×10^9/l and platelets 250×10^9/l. A repeat blood count 4 weeks later showed the same picture with a pathologist comment: 'Occasional smear cells. Marker studies may be useful to exclude a lymphoproliferative disorder'. Subsequent surface marker studies indicated coexpression of the pan-B cell antigens CD19, CD20, and HLA–DR together with CD5, CD23, and weak surface immunoglobulin with monoclonal kappa light chains. The pathologist comments 'The morphology and phenotype confirm typical B-cell chronic lymphocytic leukaemia'.

How would you advise and manage this woman?
The prognosis for this woman is excellent. She has stage A(0) disease by the International Chronic Lymphocytic Leukaemia Workshop (IWCLL) criteria and this is now the commonest presentation of the disease, with some 70 per cent of patients presenting with an asymptomatic lymphocytosis. On long-term follow-up, at least 75 per cent of such patients will have stable, non-progressive disease with a survival identical to age-matched controls. Furthermore patient subsets have been defined (using criteria such as the pattern and degree of bone marrow infiltration, total lymphocyte count $< 30 \times 10^9$/l and other criteria) where the probability of having stable, non-progressive disease is as high as 89 per cent. Unfortunately it is not possible to determine at presentation which patients will fall into the small subgroup with more aggressive disease. Females develop

chronic lymphocytic leukaemia less commonly than males (male: female ratio 2:1), and moreover have a better outlook than males as they tend to have lower stages of disease, and for each stage (A, B, or C) they less commonly progress.

No treatment is required for people with stage A chronic lymphocytic leukaemia. Indeed, there is evidence that patients treated with chlorambucil and alkylating based regimens for early-stage chronic lymphocytic leukaemia have a worse survival rate than patients who are not treated unless disease progression occurs. There is broad consensus that asymptomatic patients with only a lymphocytosis should not be treated.

Case Two: A 58-year-old man presents with 'an enlarged gland in the neck'. The patient recalls 'severe bronchitis' last winter but is otherwise well. He had what he calls 'the flu' 2 weeks ago then noticed these nodes. On physical examination you find multiple bilateral cervical nodes up to 1.5 cm diameter with numerous slightly smaller nodes in the axillae and inguinal regions. His spleen is palpable 3 cm below the costal margin and the liver edge is also palpable. FBC shows Hb 110 g/l, WBC 48×10^9/l, lymphocytes 46.5×10^9/l, and platelets 113×10^9/l. A Coombs test is negative, reticulocyte count 1.5 per cent, and ESR 25 mm/h. His biochemistry is normal but immunoglobulins are IgG 3.1, IgA 0.2, and IgM 0.1 g/l, respectively. Surface marker studies show pan-B cell antigens CD19, CD20, and HLA-DR together with CD5, CD23, and weak surface immunoglobulin with monoclonal kappa light chains. The blood film morphology and marker phenotype are typical of B-cell chronic lymphocytic leukaemia. A bone marrow trephine shows a heavy diffuse infiltrate of small lymphocytes with reduced haemopoietic reserves.

How would you advise and manage this patient?
This man has a much more significant problem than the patient discussed above with an asymptomatic lymphocytosis. He has stage B disease with lymphadenopathy and hepatosplenomegaly together with heavy marrow involvement in a diffuse pattern of infiltration resulting in impaired haemopoietic reserves. The diffuse infiltration is a poor prognostic feature although both the haemoglobin and platelets are still just above 100 g/l and 100×10^9/l respectively which are the criteria for stage C disease. The median survival for patients with stage B chronic lymphocytic leukaemia is typically about 5 to 7 years, while with stage C median survival is usually 2 to 3 years. He is panhypogammaglobulinaemic and at risk of infection, and the 'severe bronchitis' and 'flu' were probably related to his immunosuppression. Patients with advanced or progressive disease require treatment.

The patient prefers not to have treatment immediately because of work commitments and you agree to review the situation in 1 month. At this time his nodes and spleen are larger and blood count shows Hb 105 g/l, WBC 79×10^9/l with lymphocytes 77×10^9/l and platelets 105×10^9/l. However, the patient is committed to an overseas trip for work. After his return, his nodes have progressed further and he tires through the day. FBC is Hb 97 g/l, MCV 85 fl, WBC 92×10⁹/l, with lymphocytes 91×10⁹/l and platelets 85×10⁹/l. The disease is clearly progressive with a lymphocyte doubling time of < 12 months.

What should you do now?
Alkylating agents, usually chlorambucil, either with or without prednisone, have been the mainstay of treatment for many years. The drug(s) are taken orally in a variety of dosage schedules, are usually well tolerated and typically produce a good response with improvement in disease parameters (i.e. reduction in adenopathy, hepatosplenomegaly, and lymphocyte count and increase in haemoglobin and platelets) but rarely achieve criteria for complete remission. More recently, the purine analogues fludarabine and cladribine have become widely available, the former more extensively used. Both fludarabine and cladribine give an overall response rate of around 70 to 80 per cent, with around 25 to 30 per cent achieving complete remission. The purine analogues are more potently immunosuppressive and result in prolonged, severe CD4 lymphopenia which may increase the risk of infection. However, remissions achieved are usually accompanied by a good quality of life typically lasting on average 2 years before disease progression requires further therapy. Whether an alkylating agent (e.g. chlorambucil) or purine analogue (e.g. fludarabine) is most appropriate first line therapy remains controversial but may be resolved by current comparative trials.

You prescribe fludarabine 25 mg/m² intravenously on 5 consecutive days which is well tolerated. Two weeks later, the patients nodes have decreased in size and the lymphocyte count has fallen from a pretreatment level of 110×10⁹/l to 30×10⁹/l. On day 5 of his second cycle of treatment, the patient develops severe right upper abdominal pain and is admitted via the Emergency Department. He is febrile (37.5°C).

What will you do now?

Upper abdominal ultrasound and CT scan reveal a normal gall bladder, biliary tree, and pancreas, mild hepatosplenomegaly and enlarged para-aortic nodes. After 3 days, an erythematous rash appears with vesiculation and fluorescence studies confirm varicella zoster. Acyclovir and intravenous immunoglobulin are administered with prompt improvement. A fortnight later when due for treatment, he complains of increasing lethargy and appears pale. FBC showed Hb 67 g/l, MCV 110 fl, WBC 19.3×10⁹/l, lymphocytes 15.0×10⁹/l, and platelets 97×10⁹/l. The Coombs' test was positive for IgG +++ and reticulocytes were 7 per cent. Haptoglobins were low, the LDH was elevated, and bilirubin was 120 μmol/l.

The two commonest complications of chronic lymphocytic leukaemia are infection and autoimmune disease, both of which have developed here. This results in a therapeutic dilemma as the therapy of autoimmune haemolytic anaemia, namely steroids, will exacerbate the risk of infection. This is particularly the case with fludarabine and the purine analogues which are potently immunosuppressive. Furthermore, there is some evidence that purine analogues may increase the risk and severity of haemolytic anaemia. The result is that the therapeutic options for leukaemia control are reduced. For the subset of patients with hypogammaglobulinaemia and recurrent infection, intravenous immunoglobulin is effective in reducing the incidence of infection.

5.5 Myeloproliferative disorders/ myelodysplastic syndromes

A 33-year-old man presents with general malaise and tiredness for 4 months together with intense burning of his hands and feet, interfering with his ability to work. He is married with a newborn child and is under financial strain. Examination showed his hands and feet were red but otherwise normal, with a tippable spleen being the only other positive finding. FBC showed normal Hb 145 g/l, MCV 82 fl, WBC 9.2×10^9/l, with neutrophils 6.8×10^9/l and platelets 990×10^9/l.

What diagnoses would you consider in this case?
The differential diagnosis of a thrombocytosis is between primary haematological (myeloproliferative) disease and a secondary ('reactive') process. The latter include blood loss, iron deficiency, postsplenectomy state, and a wide range of acute and chronic infective and inflammatory disorders. Thrombocytosis may also occur in response to malignant disease.

Investigations reveal normal haematinic levels, including serum ferritin. The bone marrow was hypercellular involving all three haemopoietic lines with an especially marked increase in megakaryocytes. Some megakaryocytes were seen in clusters with giant and other morphologically abnormal forms. Iron stores were normal and there was no increase in reticulin. Cytogenetics show a normal male karyotype and molecular studies show absence of the *BCR/ABL* rearrangement.

What is your diagnosis and what management would you recommend?
The most likely diagnosis is essential thrombocythaemia. Essential thrombocythaemia is largely a diagnosis of exclusion and there is no specific diagnostic test. However, erythromelalgia (intense burning or throbbing pain and erythema, typically affecting the extremities) is a highly characteristic symptom of essential thrombocythaemia and results from digital microvascular ischaemia. It is usually relieved by aspirin and /or reduction of the platelet count. The decision and criteria to treat essential thrombocythaemia, especially in younger patients, is controversial. Treatment options for reduction of the platelet count include hydroxyurea, interferon, anegrelide, radioactive phosphorus (^{32}P), and perhaps other alkylating agents in occasional patients.

In younger patients, ^{32}P and alkylating agents are not acceptable because of the long-term risk of leukaemogenesis. The risks with hydroxyurea and anegrilide are low, but since younger patients may be on continuous treatment for decades these risks can accumulate to relatively high levels. There is no known risk of leukaemogenesis with interferon but it is a much more costly option. A typical starting dose would be 3 million units daily with titration against the platelet count as required. Asymptomatic patients generally do not benefit from treatment but those patients with thrombotic complications, including microvascular ischaemia, do require therapy. It is important to exclude chronic myeloid leukaemia with cytogenetics and, if possible, molecular studies (i.e. Philadelphia chromosome and *BCR/ABL* rearrangement) because of its different prognosis and management.

The patient is commenced on aspirin 300 mg/day, but continues to suffer severe symptoms. A trial of interferon is given with a fall in the platelet count but with marked and persistent side-effects. Hydroxyurea was therefore given at a continuous dose of 1 g/day. This results in a prompt fall in the platelet count and complete resolution of symptoms, with no side-effects. He remains well on hydroxyurea and aged 36, his second child was born. FBC at the time showed Hb 133 g/l, MCV 112 fl, WBC 5.2×10^9/l, neutrophils 3.2×10^9/l, and platelets 320×10^9/l. Examination was normal. (Note the macrocytosis which is particularly an effect of hydroxyurea.) Three years later, aged 39, working 15 hours a day, his third child arrived. He is asymptomatic on hydroxyurea 1 g/d. A routine follow-up FBC showed Hb 94 g/l, MCV 134 fl, WBC 3.2×10^9/l, with neutrophils 0.9×10^9/l and platelets 99×10^9/l.

What should you do now?
Pancytopaenia and more marked macrocytosis has developed on a background of previously stable essential thrombocythaemia. Hydroxyurea should be stopped and the patient should be reinvestigated.

The following results are obtained—B12 and folate levels are normal, as are routine biochemistry and liver function tests, except for an elevated LDH (750 U/l, NR 150–600 U/l). A bone marrow aspirate, trephine, and cytogenetics show trilineage myelodysplasia with blasts of 12 per cent, classified as refractory anaemia with excess blasts (RAEB) by the FAB classification. Cytogenetic analysis yields a normal male karyotype 46XY in 15 metaphases and with 46 XY, -5 in another 15 metaphases.

Tissue typing is performed on his two siblings, a younger brother, and an older sister. The sister is a fully HLA-compatible matched donor. Arrangements are made for peripheral blood stem cell (PBSC) harvesting of his HLA-compatible sister.

Following cessation of the hydroxyurea, the peripheral blood counts slowly improve and 4 weeks later the FBC show Hb 121 g/l, MCV 115 fl, WBC 4.9×10^9/l, neutrophils 2.9×10^9/l, and platelets 166×10^9/l. Examination is normal. After 6 months, the patient remains well but splenomegaly of 2 cm is noted. FBC is Hb 109 g/l, MCV 120 fl, WBC 3.5×10^9/l, neutrophils 1.8×10^9/l, and platelets 120×10^9/l. Bone marrow again shows RAEB with 15 per cent blasts. Cytogenetics now demonstrate a clone with -5, del(17p–) and –7 abnormalities in all metaphases analysed.

What do you do now?
Bone marrow transplantation is undertaken following cyclophosphamide/ busulphan conditioning using G-CSF stimulated peripheral blood stem cells harvested from his sister. Acute graft-versus-host disease develops, limited to his skin, but is controlled with cyclosporin and prednisone.

Two years later he remains alive, generally well and back at work with minor chronic graft-versus-host disease of his skin. His FBC and marrow are essentially normal with 46XX karyotype. He is planning to expand his business, and asks you what the future holds for his illness.

What do you tell him?
A relatively small proportion of patients with essential thrombocythaemia will develop acute myeloid leukaemia. Some of them may evolve into a myelodysplastic syndrome (MDS) as part of this process, as occurred in this patient. The initial finding here was the development of cytopenia with dysplastic changes in the bone marrow. The French American British (FAB) group developed a classification for MDS in 1982 based on cytopaenia, and the number of blood and marrow blasts, which was useful for prediction of prognosis as were a number of scoring systems. Equally important is the development of progressive cytogenetic abnormalities, particularly the finding of a monosomy 7 which has a particularly poor prognostic implication. The addition of cytogenetic abnormalities has improved the prognostic evaluation of myelodysplasia both with regard to survival and evolution into acute leukaemia.

5.6 A bleeding gastric carcinoma presenting as deep venous thrombosis

A previously well, 62-year-old woman presents with a 3-day history of left leg pain and swelling. On examination, there is mild left ankle oedema together with tenderness in the upper calf. Venous Doppler ultrasound demonstrates thrombus in the peroneal vein of the calf extending into the popliteal and superficial femoral veins to just below the level of the inguinal ligament. The patient is commenced on an intravenous infusion of heparin maintaining an activated partial thromboplastin time (APTT) at 1.5 to 2.5 times normal. Three days later the patient passed a large melaena, and the haemoglobin fell from 118 g/l to 78 g/l. At the time the APTT was 97 s. Because of the significant bleeding, heparin is ceased. Urgent gastroscopy reveals a 5-cm gastric carcinoma in the lower one-third of the stomach with evidence of continued bleeding.

How would you manage this patient?
This case highlights a relatively common scenario in which venous thrombo-embolic disease occurs as a complication of a malignancy. In this case the patient presents with a deep venous thrombosis as an initial manifestation of malignancy.

In the presence of a bleeding gastric cancer, treatment of an established deep venous thrombosis with full-dose, intravenous anticoagulation carries a real risk of continued and life-threatening gastrointestinal bleeding. Similarly, low molecular weight (LMW) heparin, although at least as safe and effective as standard heparin in the treatment of established venous thromboembolism (VTE), carries a similar increased risk of bleeding. Moreover, oral anticoagulants cannot be considered to be any safer than heparin, as well as having a delayed onset of action.

Accordingly, an appropriate and effective therapeutic alternative would be the insertion of an inferior vena cava (IVC) filter. This would have the advantage of preventing life-threatening embolization from the leg. It also provides time during which gastric surgery can be planned and undertaken without the attendant risk of either bleeding or pulmonary embolus. Subsequently, anticoagulation with warfarin can be instituted when the risk of bleeding is substantially less, perhaps at 1 to 2 weeks postoperatively.

VTE and cancer are linked by a two-way clinical association—VTE may be a presenting feature of occult malignancy, and patients with clinically overt cancer may develop a VTE related complication at any stage of their disease.

Patients with VTE in the absence of conventional risk factors have up to a 10 per cent likelihood of harbouring an occult cancer. However, it is not considered appropriate to subject all patients with unexplained VTE to extensive screening tests, since there is at present no evidence of a survival benefit from such a policy. Hence, it is appropriate to maintain a low threshold of suspicion of malignancy when treating patients with idiopathic VTE and to perform additional diagnostic tests only if the findings of a thorough history, physical examination, routine laboratory tests, and chest radiograph suggest the presence of a primary tumour.

Patients with cancer are at high risk of developing postoperative VTE. Hence, during periods of high risk such as surgery, they require thrombo-prophylactic measures comparable to that provided for high-risk ortho-paedic procedures. Such measures would include, for example, standard unfractionated heparin 7500 U subcutaneously twice daily, or LMW heparin, such as enoxaparin 40 mg subcutaneously daily or dalteparin 5000 U subcutaneously daily.

A number of studies have examined the risk of VTE associated with chemotherapy and central venous catheters in cancer patients. Recent data suggest a positive benefit-to-risk ratio with the systematic use of fixed mini-dose warfarin in both conditions. The only large prospective double-blind randomized study of low-dose anticoagulation in breast cancer patients demonstrated that very low-dose warfarin was an effective and safe method of prevention of thrombosis in patients with metastatic breast cancer receiving chemotherapy.

Patients with cancer who develop acute VTE should be treated with standard or LMW heparin for a minimum of 5 days. Subsequently, long-term oral anticoagulation with warfarin should be instituted to maintain the INR (International Normalized Ratio for prothrombin time) between 2 and 3, or as long as the cancer is active or chemotherapy is being given. It appears that long-term anticoagulation does not carry a significantly increased risk of major bleeding compared with the risk in patients without cancer. Although the management of patients with brain metastases or primary brain tumours should be individualized, it appears that many of these patients can be managed safely with anticoagulants. Nevertheless, anticoagulants should probably be withheld in patients with haemorrhagic brain metastases (typically those arising from melanoma or renal adeno-carcinoma), as well as those who have undergone recent craniotomies.

Cancer patients appear to carry an increased risk of recurrent thrombosis. In particular, individuals who develop a documented recurrent VTE while on oral anticoagulation represent a difficult management problem. The major options include continued warfarin except at a higher target INR, LMW heparin and IVC filter, or a combination of IVC filter and warfarin. To date, only anecdotal information exists to guide therapy in these circumstances.

There is some tantalizing data to suggest that cancer patients receiving LMW heparins may have a reduced rate of mortality. A multicentre study is currently examining the hypothesis of intrinsic antineoplastic activity of LMW heparins.

References

5.1
Mauch, P.M. (1994). Controversies in the management of early stage Hodgkin's Disease. *Blood*, **83**, 318–29.
Reuss, K., Engert, A., Tesch, H. *et al.* (1996). Current clinical trials in Hodgkin's Disease. *Annals of Oncology*, 7, 5109–5113.
Rosenberg, S.A. (1992). Reducing the toxicity of the combined modality therapy of favourable stage Hodgkin's disease. *European Journal of Cancer*, **28A**: 1379–80.
Urba, W.J. and Longo, D.L. (1992). Hodgkin's Disease. *New England Journal of Medicine*, **326**, 678–87.
5.2
Cooper, I.A., Wolf, M.M., Robertson, T.I., *et al.* (1994). Randomised comparison of MACOP-B with CHOP in patients with intermediate-grade non-Hodgkin's lymphoma. The Australian and New Zealand Lymphoma Group. *Journal of Clinical Oncology*, **12**, 769–778.
Harris, N.L., Jaffe, E.S., Stein, H., *et al.* (1994). A revised European-American classification of lymphoid neoplasms: a proposal from the International Lymphoma Study Group. *Blood*, **84**, 1361–1392.
Philip, T., Guglielmi, C., Hagenbeek, A., *et al.*, (1995). Autologous bone marrow transplantation as compared with salvage chemotherapy in relapses of

chemotherapy-sensitive non-Hodgkin's lymphoma. *New England Journal of Medicine*, **333**, 1540–1545.

5.3

Coiffier, B., Haioun, C., Ketterer, N., *et al.* (1998). Rituximab (anti-CD20 mono-clonal antibody) for treatment of patients with relapsing or refractory aggressive lymphoma. A multicenter phase II study. *Blood*, **92**, 1927–1932.

Horning, S.J. (1994).Treatment approaches to the low-grade lymphomas. *Blood*, **83**, 881–884.

Solal-Celigny, P., Lepage, E., Brousse, N., *et al.* (1996). A doxorubicin-containing regimen with or without interferon alpha 2b (IFN-2b) in advanced follicular lymphomas. Final analysis of survival, toxicity, and quality of life of the GELF 86 trial. *Blood*, **88**, 1800a.

Tallman, M.S. and Hakimian, D. (1995). Purine nucleoside analogs: emerging roles in indolent lymphoproliferative disorders. *Blood*, **86**, 2463–74.

Verdonck, L.F., Dekker, A.W., Lokhorst, E., Petersen, E.J., and Nieuwenhuis, H.K. (1997). Allogeneic versus autologous bone marrow transplantation for refractory and recurrent low-grade non-Hodgkin's lymphoma. *Blood*, **90**, 4201–4205.

Longo, D.L. (1993). What's the deal with follicular lymphomas? *Journal of Clinical Oncology*, **11**, 202–8.

5.4

Dighiero, G., Maloum, K., Desablens, B., *et al.* for French Cooperative Group on CLL (1998). Chlorambucil in chronic lymphocytic leukemia. *New England Journal of Medicine*, **338**, 1506–1514.

Mulligan, S.P. and Catovsky, D. (1993). The B-cell chronic lymphoid leukaemias. *Australian and New Zealand Journal of Medicine*, **23**, 42–50.

O'Brien, S., del Gigloi, A., and Keating, M. (1995). Advances in the biology and treatment of B-cell chronic lymphocytic leukemia. *Blood*, **85**, 307–318.

5.5

Bain, B. (1990). *Leukaemia diagnosis. A guide to the FAB classification.* Gower Medical Publishing: London.

Cunningham, I., MacCallum, S., Nicholls, M.D., *et al.* (1995). The myelo-dysplastic syndromes. An analysis of prognostic factors in 239 patients from a single institution. *British Journal of Haematology*, **90**, 602–606.

Greenberg, P., Cox, C., LeBeau, M.M., *et al.* (1997). International scoring system for evaluating prognosis in myelodysplastic syndromes. *Blood*, **89**, 2079–2088.

Schafer, A.I. (1995). Essential (primary) thrombocythemia. In *Williams hematology* (5th edn) (ed. Beutler, E., Lichtman, M.A., Coller, B.S., and Kipps, T.J.). McGraw-Hill Inc: New York.

Sterkers, Y., Preudhomme, C., La,i J.L., *et al.* (1998). Acute myeloid leukaemia and myelodysplastic syndromes following essential thrombocythaemia treated with hydroxyurea: high proportion of cases with 17p deletion. *Blood*, **91**, 616–622.

Vallespi, T., Imbert, M., Mecucci, C. *et al.* (1998). Diagnosis, classification, and cytogenetics of myelodysplastic syndromes. *Haematologica*, **83**, 258–275.

5.6

Bona, R.D., Sivjee, K.Y., and Hickey, A.D. (1995). The efficacy and safety of oral anticoagulation in patients with cancer. *Thrombosis and Haemostasis*, **74**, 1055–1058.

Levine, N.M., Hrish, J., Gent, M., *et al.* (1994). Double-blind randomized trial of very low-dose warfarin for prevention of thromboembolism in stage IV breast cancer. *Lancet*, **343**, 886–889.

Prandoni, P. (1997). Antithrombotic strategies in patients with cancer. *Thrombosis and Haemostasis*, **78**, 141–144.

Thoracic oncology

6.1 Small cell carcinoma of the lung

A 60-year-old man presents with a 4-week history of cough, and a 2-week history of dyspnoea. There is no significant past history. On direct questioning he admits to weight loss of 5 kg over 3 months. He has been a smoker of 20 cigarettes daily for 40 years. His general practitioner has performed a chest radiograph that shows a right hilar opacity, and widening of the mediastinum. Physical examination does not reveal any abnormality. Bronchoscopy is performed and a mass is seen in the right main bronchus. Biopsy of this mass is reported as showing undifferentiated small cell carcinoma.

What treatment should this man receive?
This depends on the stage of the disease. The staging system that is commonly used for small cell lung cancer (SCLC) recognizes only two stages: limited disease, defined as disease confined to one hemithorax and the ipsilateral supraclavicular lymph nodes; and extensive disease, which includes disease at any other site. The separation between limited and extensive disease has prognostic significance, with the median survival for treated patients with limited disease being approximately 18 months, while for patients with extensive disease it is approximately 12 months.

The investigations that are usually performed to stage such patients include a CT scan of the chest and upper abdomen, and a bone scan. Some clinicians also perform a CT scan of the brain. However, in the absence of neurological symptoms or signs, the yield of this investigation is low. The aim of staging investigations is to determine whether or not the patient has extensive disease. Thus, if it is apparent at the outset, either clinically or as a result of investigations, that extensive disease is present, further staging investigations may be unnecessary. Many clinical trials in SCLC also insist on a bone marrow aspirate and trephine as part of routine staging. This is not usually performed in clinical practice because of the very low yield of this test.

The results of the staging investigations indicate that the patient has disease confined to the right hemithorax, with a 4-cm mass located centrally, and mediastinal lymph nodes visible on the CT scan of the chest. On routine testing, his serum sodium was reduced, at 124 mmol/l.

How should this man be treated?

The mainstay of treatment for SCLC is now combination chemotherapy. The disease is highly responsive to many agents. The most commonly used regimens are cis- or carboplatin and etoposide (PE), or cyclophosphamide, adriamycin and vincristine (CAV). Randomized trials comparing PE to CAV have yielded identical survival for both regimens, although response rates are higher with PE. For this reason, PE, or combinations based upon it, are mostly used. Occasionally, alternating cycles of these two regimens are used; the rationale being that drug resistance may be less likely to develop. Randomized trials have not shown clear evidence of benefit with this approach, however.

Oral chemotherapy, using etoposide, either as a single agent or in combination with other drugs, has also been used to treat SCLC, particularly in elderly patients. Recent randomized trials however suggest that oral etoposide is no less toxic, less efficacious, and associated with an inferior quality of life than intravenous treatment.

With treatment, objective responses occur in 80 to 90 per cent of patients, and approximately half of these are complete responses. Treatment is usually administered for a total of six cycles (approximately 4 to 5 months). The use of maintenance chemotherapy has been investigated in randomized trials and has not been found to be of benefit.

In patients with limited SCLC treated with chemotherapy alone, the most common site of relapse is at the location of the primary tumour and associated mediastinal nodes. Radiotherapy has therefore been added to the treatment regimen for patients with limited disease. There is strong evidence from randomized trials and a meta-analysis that the addition of radiotherapy prolongs survival, with an absolute improvement of approximately 5 per cent at 5 years. The timing of radiotherapy in relation to chemotherapy is controversial, with both concurrent and sequential treatment (chemotherapy followed by radiotherapy) having been used. Although the optimal timing of radiotherapy is unclear, there are biological and clinical data to support its use as early as practical during chemotherapy. However, concurrent treatment substantially increases toxicity (especially oesophagitis), including fatal treatment-related toxicity and therefore this is reserved for good performance status patients. Because patients with extensive disease at diagnosis tend to relapse at locations other than the primary site, thoracic irradiation is not used in this group.

The optimal field size covers the gross tumour with a tight margin, as marginal recurrence is not a major pattern of failure. There is no improvement in local control above 50 Gy. Many series use hypofractionated courses of radiation, for example 40 Gy in 15 fractions, which are biologically equivalent to 50 Gy in standard 2 Gy fractions. If chemotherapy is given concurrently, the spinal cord dose is limited to 36 Gy.

The recognition that the brain may represent a sanctuary site, and therefore be a common location of relapse in patients who have achieved systemic remission, gave rise to the concept of prophylactic cranial irradiation (PCI). Patients who were responding to systemic treatment underwent cranial irradiation. Several randomized trials have shown that this approach is effective in reducing the rate of cerebral metastases, but has no impact on survival. However, individual studies of PCI were under-powered to detect a survival difference. A meta-analysis recently suggests a modest survival benefit. Initial concerns that PCI resulted in impairment of neuropsychiatric function have not been confirmed in prospective trials, which have demonstrated equivalent and relatively high rates of abnormalities in patients who received chemotherapy alone.

What is the significance of the reduced serum sodium and how should it be treated?
In this clinical context, the reduced serum sodium is likely to be a mani-festation of the syndrome of inappropriate ADH secretion. This occurs in approximately 10 per cent of cases of SCLC. There are other causes, including pulmonary inflammation and drugs. Often, the only treatment required is treatment of the underlying malignancy, since as the tumour regresses, the serum sodium usually returns to normal. However, if patients are symptomatic, or the serum sodium continues to fall, fluid restriction and demeclocycline may be required.

SCLC is also associated with other paraneoplastic manifestations, such as ectopic ACTH production, and the Eaton–Lambert myasthenic syn-drome. Although much space is often devoted to these in textbooks, they are rare, occurring in 5 per cent of cases of SCLC.

What is this patient's prognosis?
With modern treatment, the median survival for limited SCLC is approxi-mately 18 months; 5 to 15 per cent of patients are long-term survivors, and are probably cured of their disease. For patients with extensive disease, the median survival is approximately 12 months, with few long-term survivors.

If the patient responds to initial treatment but subsequently relapses, how should he be treated?
Most patients with SCLC respond to initial chemotherapy. Unfortunately most go on to relapse at a variable time following the cessation of therapy. Whether or not these patients should be treated with second-line therapy depends upon several factors, including; the duration of the remission, the drugs used initially, the site(s) of relapse, and the patient's general condition.

In patients who relapse whilst still receiving treatment, or within 3 to 6 months of completing treatment, the likelihood of a meaningful response to second-line treatment is very low. This is especially the case if their initial therapy comprised PE, since the response rate to CAV following failure of PE is 10 to 15 per cent. The converse is not true, with up to 30 per cent of patients responding to PE after failure of CAV. As a result of the limited benefit of conventional treatment, such patients ought to be considered for participation in clinical trials of new agents. When the duration of remission following initial therapy is longer (e.g. 12 to 18 months), retreatment with the same therapy as used initially is worthwhile

Short courses of radiotherapy to symptomatic disease in patients who have failed chemotherapy provide excellent rapid palliation for symptoms such as haemoptysis, cough, bone pain or cerebral metastases and is the treatment of choice for spinal cord compression and superior vena cava obstruction.

What is the role of dose intense therapy, with or without stem cell support in SCLC?
The chemoresponsiveness of SCLC has prompted many investigators to evaluate the use of higher doses or more intense programmes of chemotherapy. Although some of these approaches have yielded impressive results in single arm studies, the randomized trials that have been completed have failed to demonstrate a survival benefit. Furthermore, as might be expected, toxicity is substantially greater than with standard dose chemotherapy. However, most of the completed studies were performed before the availability of haemopoietic growth factors, current trials are re-evaluating this approach.

6.2 Non-small cell lung cancer

A 68-year-old woman presents with cough and dyspnoea. A chest radiograph reveals a peripheral left upper lobe opacity 2 cm in diameter, with widening of the mediastinum. She undergoes fine needle aspiration biopsy of the lesion, and a diagnosis of keratinizing squamous cell carcinoma is made. A CT scan of the chest and abdomen shows a left upper lobe mass but no other abnormality. Her serum calcium and alkaline phosphatase are normal

What is the optimal management for this woman?
This woman has early-stage non-small cell lung cancer (NSCLC). The optimal treatment is surgical resection. Suitability for resection depends upon her health generally and her respiratory function specifically. Sophisticated tests of respiratory function, such as differential ventilation/perfusion scanning are available, but are rarely used in practice. Assessment by a thoracic surgeon who deals commonly with lung cancer is the most appropriate method of determining suitability for surgery.

The role of mediastinoscopy in patients with early stage NSCLC is controversial. Proponents argue that the low sensitivity and specificity of CT scanning (60 to 70 per cent and 80 to 85 per cent respectively) means that the procedure is required for accurate preoperative staging. Opponents argue that the best treatment for microscopically involved nodes is surgical resection and therefore this invasive diagnostic procedure is unnecessary. The recent introduction of positron emission tomographic (PET) scanning may obviate the need for mediastinoscopy in the future.

The operation that is required depends upon the size and location of the tumour. Small peripheral lesions that do not involve the lobar fissures can usually be treated adequately by lobectomy. More central lesions or those extending across fissures are commonly treated by pneumonectomy. In patients who are unfit for a lobectomy, a wedge resection may be performed, but this procedure is associated with a higher rate of local recurrence.

The patient undergoes a left upper lobectomy and mediastinal dissection. The pathology report reveals the presence of hilar and ipsilateral mediastinal nodal involvement.

Would you recommend any adjuvant therapy?
Patients with hilar and mediastinal nodal involvement are at a higher risk of both local and distant recurrence. In recent randomized trials, post-operative radiotherapy has been shown to produce a significant reduction in local recurrence and a trend towards improved overall survival. Older randomized trials actually showed excess mortality associated with post-operative radiotherapy. As a result, institutional practices are divergent. Some radiation oncologists advise therapy for hilar disease (N1) and most give it for mediastinal disease (N2, N3) following surgery.

The dose used ranges between 40 and 60 Gy, depending on fraction size (biologically equivalent dose) and whether the identified disease was microsopic or macroscopic. The main acute toxicity is oesophagitis, which is evident towards the end of the treatment schedule and resolves slowly (over a month). The main late toxicity is lung scarring, often only evident on chest radiograph or CT. It does not usually cause major functional impairment beyond that caused by the surgery itself.

The use of adjuvant chemotherapy has also been evaluated. The data that are available are from older studies, most of which failed to show a benefit for the use of adjuvant chemotherapy. In a meta-analysis, cisplatin-containing chemotherapy was shown to produce an improvement in survival of 5 per cent at 5 years, though this was not statistically significant. Therefore, chemotherapy is not used routinely in the adjuvant setting. However, the regimens used in the individual studies that were included in the meta-analysis would not be considered optimal, and several large trials evaluating modern chemotherapy are now underway.

*What treatment would you recommend if the patient's medical condition
precluded surgical resection?*

In general, patients are judged to be medically inoperable on the basis of
severe comorbidities or advanced age. These problems often preclude the
use of combined chemoradiation or large field irradiation as well. In
clinically staged T1 and T2 lung cancer, surprisingly good results have been
reported with 'postage stamp' radiotherapy. This technique involves giving
a hypofractionated course of radiotherapy from 40 to 50 Gy in 15 to 20
fractions that gives the lesion a margin of 2 or 3 cm. The 5-year disease-free
survival is 40 per cent, but overall survival is 20 per cent as many patients
die from other illnesses.

*If mediastinal lymph node involvement had been recognized prior to surgery,
what management would you have advised?*

Management depends on the disease extent. Patients with ipsilateral
mediastinal nodes (stage IIIA) which are non-bulky are often treated with
induction or neoadjuvant chemotherapy prior to surgery. This treatment
aims to shrink the tumour to make it resectable and to control micro-
metastatic disease. Early experience suggested that this approach was relatively safe, although the possibility of a higher incidence of postoperative
complications existed. Survival was thought to be better than that in
historical controls. Further support for this approach comes from two
randomized trials, both of which compared treatment with induction
chemotherapy followed by surgery to surgery alone. In each of these
studies, survival was far better in the group treated with induction
chemotherapy, and there was no increase in postoperative complications.
There were methodological problems with these studies and further data
are awaited from recently completed trials. In the meantime, many patients
are treated with neoadjuvant chemotherapy. Typically two to three cycles of
a cisplatin-based regimen are used. Common regimens include: cisplatin
and vinorelbine; cisplatin, ifosfamide and mitomycin; and cisplatin,
vindesine and mitomycin.

Patients with bulky mediastinal nodes or stage IIIB disease (bilateral
mediastinal nodes) are not usually suitable for surgery. Those with good
performance status and <10 per cent weight loss may benefit from combined chemoradiation. The optimal sequencing of therapy is unknown and
both concurrent and neoadjuvant approaches are used. These techniques
modestly improve median survival but double 5-year survival from 10 to 20
per cent when compared with radiotherapy alone. This benefit is also seen
with radiotherapy-dose escalation alone (associated with hyperfraction-
ation, i.e. bigger dose per daily fraction size) or radiotherapy-dose intensification alone (associated with accelerated fractionation i.e. more than one
fraction per day). Logistically it is much easier to give combined modality
treatment.

Although there is no 'gold standard' chemotherapy regimen used in combined modality treatment, most reported studies have included cisplatin. Ongoing trials are evaluating the effectiveness of taxanes and other newer agents in this setting.

One year later the patient presents to her general practitioner complaining of mild nausea, left-sided chest pain, and lack of energy. Examination reveals an enlarged liver. CT scan of the abdomen shows multiple hepatic metastases, and bone scan demonstrates multiple bony metastases

What are the treatment options for this patient now?
Most patients with lung cancer present with incurable disease or relapse after attempted curative therapy and their management becomes palliative. Observation, radiotherapy, and chemotherapy all have a role.

The frail but relatively asymptomatic patient should have only supportive care. For patients with moderate-to-severe symptoms from the primary tumour, radiotherapy is the treatment of choice. Short courses of palliative radiotherapy (20 Gy in five fractions) are as effective as longer traditional courses in most cases and are preferred in terms of patient convenience and reduced toxicity. Excellent palliation is achieved for pain, cough, and bleeding. Shortness of breath and neurological problems are harder to relieve. The median time to best palliative response is 6 weeks. Retreatment of previously treated sites is worthwhile if the initial response was good and the period of palliation has been at least 6 months.

Chemotherapy has been evaluated extensively in the treatment of advanced NSCLC. Initially, questions focused on whether or not chemotherapy prolonged survival. A series of randomized trials and an associated meta-analysis have demonstrated that survival is modestly prolonged by the use of chemotherapy with an improvement in 1-year survival of 10 per cent (from 15 to 25 per cent). Opponents of the use of chemotherapy argue that this improvement is insufficient to justify the toxicity of treatment, and that treatment may have a negative influence on quality of life. This is a serious concern, given that most of the regimens used in the past have included cisplatin, and were therefore associated with nausea, vomiting, and lethargy.

Recent clinical trials which assess quality of life formally have shown that chemotherapy improves quality of life, when compared to supportive care alone. Furthermore, contemporary chemotherapy seems to be associated with better quality of life than older regimens. Further improvements might be expected with the substitution of carboplatin for cisplatin, though data from such studies are not yet available.

Notwithstanding the comments above, patient selection plays a major part in determining the outcome and tolerance of chemotherapy. Patients with poor performance status have a lower likelihood of response to chemotherapy and are more likely to experience significant side-effects.

There is no single chemotherapy regimen that has been widely accepted as a standard for use in advanced NSCLC. However, traditionally, cisplatin based regimens such as cisplatin, vindesine, and mitomycin, or cisplatin, ifosfamide, and mitomycin have been used. The recent identification of several new agents with activity in NSCLC (paclitaxel, docetaxel, gemcitabine, vinorelbine, and irinotecan) has made the choice of regimen more difficult. Numerous combinations containing these agents are currently undergoing evaluation.

6.3 Dyspnoea in a patient with lung cancer

A 65-year-old man with advanced non-small cell carcinoma of the lung has shortness of breath at rest, which becomes worse on exertion. As a result he is virtually bed-ridden, seriously impairing his quality of life.

What can be done to improve his dyspnoea?

As with any symptom management, the cause of his dyspnoea needs to be identified and reversed if possible. Recognition of reversible causes such as pulmonary embolism, bronchospasm, infection, anaemia, or effusion (either pleural or pericardial) is very important, as the palliation of irreversible causes of dyspnoea is often disappointing. A specific examination for pulsus paradoxus (a decrease in systolic arterial pressure of greater than 10 mm Hg on inspiration) should be performed, as pericardial effusion/tamponade is an underdiagnosed problem. Patients with bilateral pleural effusions commonly have pericardial effusions as well, especially in the presence of breast cancer or lung cancer.

General measures are often effective in relieving mild, intermittent dyspnoea. These include lifestyle changes and relaxation techniques. Oxygen can help, especially if the patient is hypoxic.

A variety of pharmacological agents, including opioids, have been tried for the relief of more severe dyspnoea. How opioids relieve breathlessness is uncertain. The usual explanation is that systemically administered opioids depress central respiratory centres, although it has been shown that substantial doses of morphine used for pain do not interfere with ventilatory function. Breathlessness often causes anxiety, and opioids may work largely through a central anxiolytic effect.

For the relief of breathlessness, opioids are usually administered by the conventional routes. For patients already taking morphine for pain, a 50 per cent dose increase is recommended. However, this can be problematic, since increasing the dose to control dyspnoea may aggravate side-effects such as sedation and nausea. Furthermore, the oral route depends on the patient being able to swallow, and the effect of subcutaneous morphine injection on dyspnoea is often short lived.

Various drugs used in the control of breathlessness and other respiratory symptoms can be given via a nebulizer, including normal saline, mucolytic agents, steroids, local anaesthetics, bronchodilators, and opioids. Evidence to support the efficacy of nebulized morphine is limited. A retrospective chart review claimed that nebulized opioid treatment was effective in >70 per cent of cases with breathlessness due to malignant disease, and a small uncontrolled prospective study found reductions in breathlessness that were maintained for 48 hours. However, of four controlled trials in patients with chronic obstructive lung disease, only one found that nebulized morphine was effective. The only controlled study of nebulized morphine in patients with advanced cancer also failed to confirm an advantage for nebulized morphine. Dosages and schedules of nebulized morphine are largely empirical, a starting dose of 20 mg being advocated with doses up to 100 mg being used. Although it has been postulated that inhaled morphine relieves breathlessness through a local action in the lung, this is controversial.

Nebulized drugs are not without their drawbacks. Some patients cannot tolerate wearing a mask; a mouthpiece may be better tolerated. Nebulized morphine can occasionally induce bronchospasm due to histamine release, so the first dose should be given under careful supervision. Maintaining equipment without the support of a respiratory therapy service can be a practical consideration when using nebulized morphine in the community.

6.4 Delirium in a patient with lung cancer

A 64-year-old man has non-small cell lung cancer and multiple bone metastases, which were present at the time of diagnosis. He has been treated palliatively with radiotherapy. His family complains that he 'has not been himself' the last few days. Last night he asked to speak to his wife who has been dead for 2 years.

How would you assess this patient?
This man has a delirium, a diagnosis that can only be made clinically. Delirium represents a loss of the brain's ability to integrate and control information. It is always due to a serious physical assault on cerebral function, and is a clear sign the patient is very unwell. Its core feature is a fluctuating inability to shift, sustain, and focus attention. Generally the patient will appear vague, perplexed, or confused. Emotional lability is a common feature. Less commonly the patient may suffer delusions and auditory or visual hallucinations. Few will misdiagnose the floridly delirious patient who is agitated and responding to frightening visual hallucinations. In milder cases though, the patient may appear quiet or withdrawn. These cases are often overlooked or mistaken for anxiety or depression. As delirium is usually worst at night, the daytime diagnosis of a mild delirium is particularly difficult.

Any patient in whom mental changes are noted should receive some formal cognitive testing. Ask the patient if he knows where he is and if he knows the day, date, and year. Ask him to remember five words and test his recall immediately and at two minutes. Finally test the patient's concentration by asking him to recite the months of the year in reverse order. Record not only the answers the patient gives, but also how far off wrong answers were. To think it is Wednesday when it is actually Thursday is unlikely to be significant, but to think that it is December when it is actually March will be.

How should this man be managed?
The management of delirium is two fold. First, find and reverse the underlying medical problem, then control any behavioural disturbance as appropriate. Most episodes of delirium will have more than one medical cause. Any acute pathophysiological disturbance can contribute to a delirium. In this patient, likely contributors would include respiratory infection, hypoxia, electrolyte disturbances such as hypercalcaemia, side-effects of analgesia, and the effects of possible cerebral secondaries. The clinician should search for the underlying medical cause, perform investigations as clinically appropriate, and then reverse the disturbances as far as possible.

Behavioural problems associated with a delirium will often respond to simple measures, such as repeated reassurance or soft lighting. If, however, the patient is extremely distressed or the behaviour is jeopardizing management, temporary chemical sedation may be warranted. In these cases, haloperidol in doses of 0.5 to 2.0 mg at night, or twice a day, is the drug of choice. Haloperidol is subject to extensive first pass metabolism by the liver. In patients with disordered liver function, a reduced dosage schedule should be considered. Generally a delirium will resolve within a week or so of the acute disturbance being normalized.

6.5 Seizures in a patient with lung cancer and cerebral metastases

A 48-year-old woman with lung cancer has a 'funny turn' while shopping in a supermarket. She is brought to the emergency department and a cerebral CT scan shows multiple brain metastases. A chest radiograph shows a hilar opacity. How should this woman be managed?

A tissue diagnosis of malignancy must be obtained from the chest lesion before making a diagnosis of multiple cerebral metastases.

Patients with far advanced cancer may be subject to 'funny turns' for several reasons. It is important to differentiate focal or generalized seizures from widespread myoclonus of an opioid or metabolic origin, localized muscle spasm, or syncopal episodes (particularly due to postural hypotension).

A generalized tonic–clonic convulsion beginning with localized fitting in an area neurologically corresponding to a known metastasis is relatively certain ground. However, a first, generalized convulsion in a patient with ataxia due to a cerebral metastasis who has had a recent fall and bumped their head may be due to subdural haematoma.

Medications (both prescribed and otherwise) should also be reviewed, looking for drugs that may lower the fitting threshold (e.g. neuroleptics), or recent withdrawal of drugs (e.g. benzodiazepines and alcohol). Morphine in very high doses may cause generalized convulsions as well as the more commonly recognized myoclonus.

The seizure is attributed to the metastatic disease in this case. What treatment options are available?

Measures to reduce oedema associated with cerebral metastases (dexamethasone 4 to 8 mg twice a day) may be useful. Radiotherapy is the main anticancer modality used, although not all patients will benefit from cerebral irradiation. Its antiepileptic effect seems to extend beyond tumour reduction. Chemotherapy might be considered if the primary tumour were small cell carcinoma. Occasional patients with a solitary cerebral metastasis, and without rapidly progressive systemic disease, might benefit from surgical metastasectomy, if the tumour is located in a surgically favourable region.

For the urgent treatment of fitting, options depend on the setting and the available means of administration. Intravenous diazepam 5 to 10 mg (or another benzodiazepine—midazolam, clonazepam, lorazepam) is appropriate in the hospital setting. Elsewhere, rectal diazepam 10 mg (using the intravenous formulation rather than a suppository), or subcutaneous midazolam 2.5 to 5 mg may be more practical. Repeated doses may be necessary, the upper dosage limit being determined by apparent effectiveness, respiratory effort, and degree of sedation. If multiple fits occur within a short period, it is prudent to start a subcutaneous infusion. Uncommonly, benzodiazepines are ineffective and consideration should be given to an intravenous infusion of phenytoin (under close monitoring for arrhythmia, bradycardia, or hypotension) or a stat dose of phenobarbitone 100 to 200 mg by intramuscular injection followed by a subcutaneous infusion of phenobarbitone 200 to 600 mg/day. This drug has a long half-life and can be very sedating.

For recurrent fitting, maintenance therapy with standard anticonvulsants is usual therapy. Carbamazepine and valproate can be continued rectally in patients unable to take oral medications. Clonazepam (sublingual or subcutaneous) can be substituted. The dose is variable (1 to 6 mg/day) and is titrated against efficacy and sedation. The sublingual route may be ineffective for a patient with a dry mouth. Midazolam can also be given by subcutaneous infusion, the dose (10 to 60 mg/day) being adjusted in a similar way.

Carers often express great concern about the possibility of fitting in a patient with cerebral metastases who is cared for at home. They need to recognize a true seizure and understand what immediate action is necessary. Carers may be instructed in the use of subcutaneous midazolam, the urgent use of which is made easier by a subcutaneous catheter already being in place.

6.6 Metallic stent for superior vena cava obstruction in a patient with far advanced lung cancer*

A 75-year-old woman has a past history of cancer of the right breast 25 years previously, treated by mastectomy and axillary clearance followed by extensive radiotherapy. Subsequently she has remained well until 1 year ago, when she had an episode of haemoptysis. Chest radiograph and CT scan at the time showed a large mass in the upper lobe of the right lung, infiltrating into the adjacent anterior chest wall and superior mediastinum. Biopsy of the mass confirmed adenocarcinoma but it was uncertain whether this was a second primary lung cancer or a late metastasis from her previous breast cancer. No further radiotherapy could be offered because of her past treatment, so she was treated with tamoxifen and then medroxyprogesterone in the hope it was metastatic breast cancer. The haemoptysis resolved on this regimen although the mass did not shrink. The patient now presents with the symptoms and signs of superior vena cava (SVC) obstruction, including shortness of breath at rest, stridor, and distention of the neck veins, developing over a few weeks. Chest radiograph shows the right lung mass to be larger.

What treatment options are available in this case?
Management of malignancy-associated SVC obstruction presents a complex clinical challenge. SVC obstruction occurs in several contexts, requiring different treatment approaches; as the presenting problem in newly diagnosed patients, as a thrombotic complication of central vascular access in patients receiving chemotherapy, and as manifestation of progressive disease in patients with advanced cancer, such as in this case.

Given time, collateral circulation can develop in patients with advanced disease and the symptoms resolve spontaneously, so no treatment may be

* Reprinted by permission of Elsevier Science from N. Young and P. Glare (in press). Case Report: use of a metallic stent for symptom relief of superior vena caval obstruction in a patient with advanced cancer. *Journal of Pain and Symptom Management*.

needed if the symptoms are mild. In patients with distressing symptoms, there are various options. Radiotherapy, chemotherapy, and/or cortico-steroids may all be effective. Radiotherapy is initially successful in over 90 per cent of cases, although there is a 20 per cent recurrence rate (due to such factors as tumour regrowth, radiation fibrosis, and caval thrombosis). Unfortunately, this patient had previously had maximal radiotherapy, so no more could be given. Chemotherapy was not offered because it was considered to be unlikely to palliate her symptoms quickly enough and would cause substantial toxicity. Surgery is no longer considered to have a role. Dexamethasone was therefore tried (8 mg/day), and provided a good symptom response within 48 hours. She was discharged home on a dose of 4 mg/day, which was to be maintained subsequently.

The patient re-presents 6 weeks later with progressive symptoms and is very distressed. There is no response after 48 hours to an increase in the dexamethasone dose (to 8 mg/day again).

What can be done now?
Re-establishment of the SVC lumen with metal stents is now advocated when conventional therapy has failed and symptoms recur. This technique was first reported in 1986, and improvements in stent technology and delivery application now allows highly accurate and simple delivery placement systems. A high rate of success in stent placement and lumen recannalization is therefore expected, with rapid resolution of symptoms. Complication rates for the procedure are low—thrombosis, stent misplacement, and migration being the main problems. Survival time postprocedure is short, however, around 3 to 6 months in most series.

Right arm venography and SVC venography showed a high grade stenosis of the SVC caused by tumour encasement and infiltration. A metal self-expanding stent was placed successfully across the stricture, with assistance by intraluminal balloon angioplasty. Postprocedure, the symptoms improved dramatically, with resolution of her stridor and improved shortness of breath within 24 hours. There was also objective reduction in head, neck, and arm swelling in the following days. The procedure entailed no complications, and the patient returned home, well palliated, 6 days later.

Over the next few weeks, the patient began to lose weight and became increasingly weak. She was admitted to an inpatient hospice unit where she died a short time later, exactly 1 month after stent insertion. The symptoms did not recur during this time. You are asked to justify the use of this expensive, invasive procedure to the hospital's Patient Care Committee.

What case will you make to justify your decision?
Interventional radiology, such as stenting of the SVC, is increasingly being offered to cancer patients, but there is much disagreement about their

appropriateness in patients with far advanced disease. On the one hand, these procedures are expensive and challenge the traditional non-technological paradigm of palliative care, but on the other hand they are minimally invasive and can have an immediate and dramatic positive impact on quality of life in appropriately selected patients, particularly when simpler approaches have been ineffective.

The process of clinical decision-making regarding patient selection for the use of modern medical technology in the setting of far advanced cancer is complex. Many factors need to be taken into account, including:

(1) clinical details (tumour type, extent of disease, natural history, previous treatments, prognosis);
(2) the risks and harms to the patient of the intervention;
(3) the benefit to the patient of the intervention;
(4) the patient's goals, priorities, and expectations at this stage of their illness;
(5) future management problems if the intervention is/is not performed;
(6) ethical and legal issues (including cost).

This calculus, which is part of any clinical decision making, is more complicated in patients with advanced disease; benefits must clearly outweigh risks to justify an intervention, yet these are all difficult to measure with any certainty in the terminal stages when outcomes are mainly subjective and the clinical status of the patient is deteriorating rapidly. Patient preference may also change rapidly, as the goal of treatment changes.

Why was the decision made in this patient the correct one?
Prior to the development of the SVC obstruction, her cancer followed a relatively indolent course and she was maintaining a good performance status with few symptoms. Although she only survived 1 month post-procedure, her prognosis had been estimated to be around 3 months, with a small chance of lasting up to a year. Her level of symptomatic distress did not allow us to manage her conservatively, however, even though it was judged that there would probably be enough time for a collateral circulation to develop.

The burden of the procedure was perceived to be small and the benefits large for this particular patient. The patient understood what the procedure involved, our uncertainty about its outcome in her case, and our belief that serious side-effects were unlikely. Without the intervention, she believed her symptoms would worsen before spontaneous resolution occurred. As a result, she had absolutely no hesitation in submitting herself for the procedure.

The fact that the patient lived only 1 month after the procedure may have been disappointing from a cost-effectiveness point of view, but only served to vindicate the decision to intervene rather than wait. We believe the cost of the intervention (approximately $A 4000) was justified in this case. The patient was very satisfied with the outcome in terms of the rapidity of symptom control and the minimal burden involved, and we believed her prognosis was still measured in terms of months when we performed it. Those who administer health funds might view this decision differently, however.

References

6.2

Ginsberg, R.J., Rubinstein, L.V., for the Lung Cancer Study Group (1995). Randomized trial of lobectomy versus limited resection for T1 NO non-small cell lung cancer. *Annals of Thoracic Surgery*, **60**, 615–22.

Rossell, R., Gomez-Codina, J. Camps, C. *et al.* (1994). A randomized trial comparing preoperative chemotherapy plus surgery with surgery alone in patients with non-small cell lung cancer. *New England Journal of Medicine*, **330**, 153–158.

Roth, J.A., Fosella, F., Komaki, R. *et al.* (1994). A randomized trial comparing perioperative chemotherapy and surgery with surgery alone in resectable stage III A non-small cell lung cancer. *Journal of the National Cancer Institute*, **86**, 673–680.

6.3

Ahmedzai, S. and Davis, C. (1997). Nebulised drugs in palliative care. *Thorax*, **52** Suppl 2, S75–7.

Booth, S., Kelly, M.J., Cox, N.P. *et al.* (1996). Does oxygen help dyspnoea in patients with cancer? *American Journal of Respiratory and Critical Care Medicine*, **153**, 1515–8.

Boyd, K.J. and Kelly, M. (1997). Oral morphine as symptomatic treatment of dyspnoea in patients with advanced cancer. *Palliative Medicine*, **11**, 277–81.

Walsh, D. (1993). Dyspnoea in advanced cancer. *Lancet*, **342**, 450–1.

6.4

Lipowski, Z.J. (1987). Delirium (acute confusional states). *Journal of the American Medical Association*, **258**, 1789–1792.

Lishman, W.A. (1998). *Organic psychiatry. The psychological consequences of cerebral disorder*. Blackwell Science: London.

Trzepacz, P.T. (1996). Delirium. Advances in diagnosis, pathophysiology and treatment. *Psychiatric Clinics of North America*, **19**, 429–448.

6.6

Oudkerk, M., Kuijpers, T.J., Schmitz, P.I. *et al.* (1996). Self-expanding metal stents for palliative treatment of superior vena caval syndrome. *Cardiovascular and Interventional Radiology*, **19**, 146–51.

Thomson, K.R. (1997). Interventional radiology. *Lancet*, **350**, 354–8.

Tuch, H. and Woodrow, A. (1995). Technology in terminal illness. *Journal of Palliative Care*, **11** (absract), 68.

7

Urological oncology

7.1 Testicular carcinoma

A 25-year-old male ambulance driver presents with a 4-day history of facial twitching. He has been otherwise well and has no past history of significant illnesses. On examination he looks fit and healthy. Neurological examination is normal. General examination is normal except that his right testis is small and hard. A cerebral CT scan shows a solitary enhancing lesion in the right temporal lobe with surrounding oedema. Plain chest radiograph shows a right lower lobe lesion. Chest and abdominal CT scans show the right lower lobe lung lesion (5 × 6 cm) as well as a 3 × 4-cm para-aortic node mass in the abdomen. Serum α-fetoprotein (AFP) is elevated to 295 and β-human chorionic gonadotrophin (β-HCG) to 550. Cerebrospinal fluid (CSF) cytology and biochemistry are normal.

What is the likely diagnosis?
The patient probably has metastatic germ cell tumour of the testis. He will need multimodality treatment to optimize the chance of cure, but the prognosis is poor.

How would you manage this problem?
The patient should be commenced on dexamethasone and phenytoin whilst definitive therapy is arranged. His brain metastasis requires urgent therapy. Patients with germ cell tumours presenting with brain metastases have a better prognosis than those patients who develop brain metastases after initial treatment (i.e. in the setting of chemotherapy-resistant disease). The standard treatment is surgical excision if possible, followed by whole brain radiotherapy and chemotherapy. Choriocarcinoma metastases, in particular, have a marked propensity for intracerebral bleeding if initially treated with chemotherapy without surgery.

At the same time, he should have a bilateral testicular ultrasound and if a primary tumour is found, this should be treated by radical inguinal orchidectomy. This should be done despite the presence of metastatic disease since:

- it will give a histological diagnosis;
- it will determine whether mature teratoma is present which may have implications for later resection of a residual mass;

- the testis is a sanctuary site protected from chemotherapy—chemotherapy may not completely eradicate cancer in the testis despite completely clearing metastatic sites.

The patient's ultrasound demonstrates a small right testis containing areas of calcification consistent with tumour. An inguinal orchidectomy is performed and histology reveals predominantly embryonal cell carcinoma with some areas of yolk sac tumour.

He will require cisplatin based chemotherapy followed by resection of any residual masses at the completion of chemotherapy. Standard chemotherapy is *b*leomycin, *e*toposide, and cis*p*latinum (i.e. BEP).

The patient was commenced on BEP chemotherapy, and also received granulocyte-colony stimulating factor (G-CSF) daily by subcutaneous injection on days 6 to 16. During the first cycle of BEP, the patient experienced no emesis but moderate nausea towards the end of the first week of treatment. There were no other problems. On day 1 of cycle 2 the blood count results were: leucocyte count $1.2 \times 10^9/l$, neutrophils $0.5 \times 10^9/l$, haemoglobin 120 g/dl, platelets $110 \times 10^9/l$. He is otherwise well and afebrile.

Should his next treatment be delayed in the presence of neutropenia?
The answer is definitely NO!

Treatment delays increase the likelihood of emergence of drug-resistant tumour cells. Treatment should proceed on schedule in full dosage.

Treatment was given on time and in full dosage, and his serum tumour markers fell to normal levels. At the completion of four cycles of chemotherapy there was a 2×1-cm residual mass in the left lower lobe of the lung and a 3×2-cm residual left para aortic node persisting on CT scan.

What should be done now?
There is some variability in opinion as to which patients should undergo surgical resection of residual masses after chemotherapy. A residual mass after chemotherapy may contain viable cancer, and standard management in most centres is to resect such masses. Surgery alone may be curative in this setting, but if viable tumour is found most centres advise further chemotherapy. If the mass is thought to be technically unresectable, radiotherapy may be an option for treatment of residual masses.

Another difficulty is where patients have residual disease in both the chest and abdomen and therefore would need two procedures for resection. Patients should first have a retroperitoneal resection and if this reveals only necrotic tissue it is reasonable to observe the pulmonary lesions, particularly where the pulmonary resection would be difficult.

Young patients may develop thymic hyperplasia on chemotherapy, and this should not be mistaken for residual tumour mass after therapy.

Are there any other issues to consider before embarking upon surgical resection?
Yes!

After bleomycin therapy, exposure to high inspired oxygen tensions during anaesthesia has been associated with severe and even fatal pneumonitis. The anaesthetist must be aware that the patient has received bleomycin therapy, and should ensure that the inspired oxygen tension remains no more than 24 per cent if at all possible. Under these conditions, development of pneumonitis is rare.

Both masses are resected during the one operative procedure. Histology shows mostly necrotic tissue with one area of mature teratoma in the pulmonary mass. No further treatment was given. The patient recovered well from the procedure.

How should this man be followed up? What investigations should be performed; how often and for how long?
The single most important routine test leading to diagnosis of relapse is serum AFP and HCG, even if the patient was previously marker negative. Regular clinical examination, chest radiograph, and abdominopelvic CT scan are of little value, particularly if the immediate post treatment scans were normal. For non-seminoma germ cell tumours, 90 per cent of relapses occur within 2 years. Late relapsing cancers have a different biology to those relapsing early and surgery is the preferred mode of therapy.

Patients with testicular carcinoma have an increased incidence of contralateral primary tumours. Such new primaries may cause a rise in serum tumour markers and masquerade as a distant relapse of the initial tumour.

In this patient, initial postoperative CT scans of the brain, chest, abdomen, and pelvis are normal. The planned follow-up is for clinic visits every 2 months for the first year, every 3 months during the second year, every 4 months during the third year, 6-monthly for the fourth and fifth year, and then yearly afterwards indefinitely. On each visit he will have a clinical examination and blood taken for AFP and BHCG.

7.2 Options to preserve fertility after treatment for testis cancer

A 28-year-old male with a testicular germ cell tumour undergoes a right orchidectomy, and is about to receive chemotherapy and/or radiotherapy which is expected to cause azoospermia. He wishes to retain the possibility of being able to father a child.

What are the options to preserve his fertility?
All postpubertal males should be given the option of having sperm cryo-stored prior to receiving sterilizing doses of chemotherapy or radiotherapy.

It is intended these samples be used for intrauterine insemination of his partner. The duration of cryostorage does not appear to alter the quality of the frozen sperm. Several samples should be collected by masturbation with a period of 3 to 5 days between collections.

Unfortunately the number and quality of semen samples obtained prior to cancer therapy are often unsatisfactory for use in standard intrauterine insemination procedures. In addition, the process of freezing and thawing sperm may reduce their density and motility. In this situation, fertilization may be achieved by *in vitro* fertilization of aspirated oocytes (IVF). This requires that the patient's partner complete a cycle of controlled ovarian hyperstimulation to allow collection of several mature oocytes.

Intracytoplasmic injection of a single sperm (ICSI) was first used to achieve fertilization in 1992. Several thousand babies have now been born using this procedure to cause fertilization. When ejaculated sperm are not available, the possibility of obtaining sperm by direct percutaneous aspiration of the epididymis or testis should be considered. Viable immature spermatozoa or spermatids obtained in this manner may be cryostored for use after thawing in the ICSI procedure. The probability of being able to obtain sperm by percutaneous aspiration is best correlated with the volume and consistency of the testis.

Animal experiments with testicular implants have demonstrated survival of Sertoli cells and androgen-producing interstitial cells. Although germ cells are more vulnerable to ischaemia in implants, a few have survived in immature grafts and were able to undergo maturation. This means that for patients requiring therapy which may destroy the testis, it is possible that small segments of seminiferous tubule isolated by testicular biopsy could be cryopreserved then autografted after completion of cancer therapy. This technique may be useful in prepubertal boys in whom sperm are not available. Alternatively, fertility may be restored in future treatments by cryostorage then transfer of isolated spermatogonial stem cells.

7.3 Prostate cancer

A 63-year-old man presents after watching a television documentary on prostate cancer. He asks for 'a PSA test to check for prostate cancer'.

What is prostate specific antigen (PSA)?
PSA is a normal protein found in the prostate and seminal vesicles. Its function is to maintain semen in the liquid state, essential for fertility. PSA can also degrade the extracellular matrix, and it has been hypothesized that PSA may have a role in the development of metastases in prostatic carcinoma. Despite the use of the word 'specific' in its name, PSA mRNA has been detected in many tissues other than the prostate, including kidney,

pituitary, endometrium, and breast. It is even found in very low levels in female serum. However, for practical purposes, only diseases of the prostate cause an elevation of serum PSA as measured by currently available assays. PSA levels can be elevated by any prostate disease, including prostatitis, benign prostatic hypertrophy, and prostate cancer.

PSA is a member of the kallikrein family, of which there are three members—KLK1, 2, and 3. PSA is KLK2. KLK1 plays a role in the normal haemostatic/coagulation process. The role of KLK3 is unknown.

The normal serum PSA level correlates with age and prostate volume. Prostatic manipulations (e.g. digital rectal examination, transrectal ultrasound) do not produce clinically significant elevations of serum PSA. Transurethral resection or prostatic biopsy do elevate PSA levels significantly. The enzyme prostatic acid phosphatase was used extensively prior to the advent of PSA measurement. Prostatic acid phosphatase has been replaced by PSA measurement because of technical difficulties with cross-reactivity in assays, and the fact that manipulation of the prostate can significantly alter serum acid phosphatase levels.

How useful is measuring serum prostate specific antigen (PSA) as a screening test for prostate cancer?

Screening programmes for cancer target a population of apparently healthy people without symptoms or signs of illness (Case 1.10). The aim is to detect disease at an early stage with the goal of reducing subsequent morbidity and/or mortality. In apparently healthy men who are ultimately diagnosed as having prostate cancer, PSA levels rise some years prior to ultimate diagnosis. In men ultimately found to have metastatic disease, this rise in PSA commences 5 to 10 years prior to the time of diagnosis. This data would imply that there is a 5 to 10-year lead time on a clinical diagnosis of prostate cancer, within which a screened population of asymptomatic men could undergo early detection of potentially curable cancers. However, this data also suggests that the value of detecting early cancers in men with an expected survival of only 5 to 10 years may be limited.

There are several ways in which the concept of PSA screening for prostate cancer fails to fulfil the requirements for a successful programme (see Case 1.10). In particular, the reported incidence of prostate cancer has risen dramatically over the last decade. This is thought to reflect, in large part, the widespread availability of the PSA blood test, which has enabled detection of cancers which would not otherwise have been clinically diagnosed. If the increasing incidence of prostate cancer was due entirely to the fact that more men were developing prostate cancer, then the mortality, and disease-specific mortality, would be expected to rise, but this has not occurred. A proportion of these cancers may never have become life threatening, and the patient may have died of other causes without the cancer ever being diagnosed. Autopsy series examining the incidence of prostate cancer support this view. It has been estimated that the lifetime risk of a healthy 50-year-old man developing a clinical cancer is just under 10 per cent, which is approximately one-quarter the chance of having a cancer found in the prostate at the time of death (i.e. an autopsy cancer). Even if cancer is detected clinically in the hypothetical 50-year-old man at some point in his subsequent lifetime, his risk of dying from prostate cancer, rather than from another cause, is less than 3 per cent. Data such as these would tend to support the concern that prostate cancer has a potential for being 'overdiagnosed', thus leading to unnecessary, and potentially harmful, investigations or treatments. More sophisticated screening approaches, including combinations of digital rectal examination, transrectal ultrasound, and PSA are under investigation.

In response to direct questioning, the patient states that no-one in his family has been diagnosed with prostate cancer, but his mother and sister had been treated for breast cancer, and an aunt died of ovarian cancer.

What is the significance of this family history?
A family history of prostate cancer occurs in 10 per cent of cases. The relative risk of prostate cancer for a male with a first degree relative with prostate cancer is 1.76, that is the risk is 76 per cent higher among first degree relatives of prostate cancer patients compared to first degree relatives of controls. The risk increases with the number of relatives affected and with younger age of onset. For example for a male with three or more cases in the family and one case developing under the age of 65 years, the relative risk for prostate cancer is 4 to 14 fold. Genetic analysis of kindreds with very high incidence of prostate cancer suggests the existence of a dominantly inherited high-risk gene (*prostate cancer* susceptibility gene— *PRCA1*), but this gene has not yet been identified.

Inherited mutations in the tumour suppressor genes *BRCA1* and *BRCA2*, which confer a high risk of breast and ovarian cancer in females, also confer a three-fold increased risk of prostate cancer in male family members who carry the gene mutation (see Cases 1.2 and 3.1).

On questioning, the patient gives a 6-month history of poor urine flow, urinary frequency, and five episodes of nocturia each night. General examination is normal. Rectal examination reveals a moderately enlarged prostate which is firm, but no nodules are felt. The lateral and median prostatic sulci are palpable. His PSA level is found to be 30.2 ng/ml.

What is the significance of this result and what should be done now?
The higher the serum PSA level above the age-specific range, the greater the chance of having prostate cancer on biopsy. The patient should undergo transrectal ultrasound, and sextant biopsies (a systematic series of six

biopsies, three from each lobe) as well as specific biopsy of any abnormality detected on ultrasound.

The pathology report from sextant biopsies describes three out of six biopsies containing poorly differentiated adenocarcinoma, Gleason Grade 4 + 5, (Gleason Score 9).

How would you manage the patient now?
The Gleason system is the most commonly used histological grading system. This assigns a grade (1 being well differentiated through to 5 for poorly differentiated) for both the primary and secondary growth patterns of the tumour. The two numbers are combined to give a score out of 10. The higher the score, the greater the probability of extracapsular spread and nodal metastasis. A number of algorithms exist whereby the Gleason score, clinical tumour staging, and PSA levels are combined to predict the likelihood of disease spread beyond the prostate.

Before embarking on radical therapy (either radical surgery or radical irradiation), regional nodes are usually assessed radiologically or by laparoscopic sampling. Patients with any lymph node metastases have a greater than 80 per cent probability of tumour recurrence within 10 years regardless of therapy, and a two to three fold higher risk of dying of prostate cancer within 10 years compared to those without node involvement.

A bone scan should be performed if the PSA level is higher than 20 ng/ml, or if bone symptoms are present.

Bone scan is normal, and four obturator nodes removed at laparoscopy are free of tumour.

What are the management options now?
There are often valid alternatives for management of localized prostate cancer. The decision as to how best to treat a particular man is influenced by:

- Patient factors—a man's age, general fitness, and concurrent medical problems, and the patient's preference once he has been fully appraised of the options.
- Tumour factors—tumour stage, Gleason score, and pretreatment PSA level may preclude one or more forms of treatment. For example radical prostatectomy would not be appropriate for a tumour not localized to the gland. Treatment with curative intent may not be appropriate if the PSA is very high, regardless of clinical stage.
- Treatment factors—it is important to consider morbidity profiles of surgery and radiation therapy as well as the geographic accessibility of treatment options.

Tumours confined to the prostate are generally managed by radical surgery or irradiation. In some cases 'watchful waiting' or deferred therapy is preferable. There are no definitive, prospective, randomized trials of comparably staged patients treated with radical surgery versus radical irradiation, so that there is no evidence for superiority of any therapy. Comparing outcomes in non-randomized surgical and radiation therapy series is problematic because of significant differences in patient populations (e.g. pathologically staged patients in surgical series versus clinically staged patients in radiation series, generally fitter patients in surgical series, etc.) and the fact that radiation series often include greater numbers of more advanced tumours.

Reported complication types and rates for each modality vary considerably. Causes for this variability include the experience of the centre, case selection, and variation in definitions used to describe toxicities and their severity. Relevant endpoints include acute morbidity/mortality and longer-term complications such as urinary incontinence, lack of potency, and potential injury to bladder and rectum. Information given to patients should, wherever possible, include the local experience of morbidity, rather than that reported by other centres.

The patient chooses to undergo radical prostatectomy. Histopathology on the resected specimen shows Gleason grade 4 + 5 adenocarcinoma with a positive surgical margin. There are no immediate postoperative complications. The urinary catheter is removed on day 5. However, the patient remains incontinent of urine requiring four pads per day.

Should the patient receive postoperative radiotherapy?
Maybe!

The routine combination of prostatectomy and postoperative radiation therapy is not of proven benefit, although trials addressing this question are in progress. Late morbidity of radiation is increased following surgery, and delay of pelvic irradiation until continence is regained is advisable if treatment is to be given. Possible indications include microscopic capsular breach (not suspected prior to surgery) and/or tumour involvement of surgical margins. However, only about one in three patients with prostatectomy margins reported as positive go on to manifest evidence of locoregional progression. In addition, the definition of 'involved' or 'equivocal' margins is controversial.

The potential survival benefit of adjuvant radiotherapy is limited to patients who are at low risk of having distant metastases or regional spread to lymph glands; thus seminal vesicle involvement, known node involvement, and/or a serum PSA that does not fall postoperatively to normal should be considered contraindications to the use of postoperative radiotherapy.

7.4 Renal cell carcinoma with intracaval extension

A 54-year-old man has been generally unwell for some 12 months. His family physician documented moderate normocytic normochromic anaemia 6 months ago, but the patient has refused further investigation. He is hypertensive with mild chronic airflow limitation. On prompting from his family the patient undergoes a CT scan of the abdomen which demonstrates a large solid mass in the right kidney with extension into the inferior vena cava up to the level of the hepatic veins.

What is the most likely diagnosis?

A solid tumour with extension into the inferior vena cava (IVC) is most likely a primary renal cell carcinoma, but occasionally other tumours may extend into the renal vein or IVC. These include transitional cell or squamous cell carcinoma of the renal pelvis and renal sarcoma.

What further investigations are recommended?

- Urea, electrolytes and creatinine, full blood count and liver function tests;
- chest radiograph;
- MRI or cavogram.

Caval tumour extension has traditionally been delineated with an inferior cavogram. Usually performed via a femoral vein puncture, this approach may not demonstrate the superior extent of the tumour thrombus well. A superior cavogram may be necessary. Magnetic resonance imaging (MRI) is as sensitive at detecting IVC tumour thrombus as vena cavography but has no risk of dislodging thrombus, and has become the investigation of choice. Spiral CT scan with reconstruction may give similar results.

Bone scan is only indicated if there is any suspicion of bony metastasis such as bone pain or abnormal alkaline phosphatase.

What paraneoplastic syndromes are known to be associated with renal cell carcinoma?

- polycythaemia;
- anaemia;
- hypercalcaemia;
- hypocalcaemia;
- pyrexia of unknown origin (PUO);
- Staiffer syndrome (abnormal liver function tests without demonstrable liver secondaries);
- elevated erythrocyte sedimentation rate (ESR);
- polyneuropathy;
- diabetes mellitus.

What are the treatment options and prognosis?
Despite advances in radiotherapy, chemotherapy, and immunotherapy, renal cell carcinoma remains a surgical disease. Complete excision (radical nephrectomy) is the only effective treatment. Prognosis depends on pathological stage of the tumour. This patient has a 70 per cent chance of surviving 5 years if the lymph nodes are not involved.

The presence of caval tumour thrombus does not alter prognosis as long as all tumour is removed. Prognosis is poor in the presence of lymph node involvement.

7.5 Transitional cell carcinoma of the mid-ureter in a patient with only one kidney

A 72-year-old male presents for follow-up after recently moving into the region. The patient underwent a left nephroureterectomy 5 years ago for transitional cell carcinoma (TCC) of the left kidney. Six months ago 'follow-up' cystoscopy had shown a large superficial TCC in the right ureter which had been completely resected. His general health was good for his age but he had poor vision and mild dementia.

What investigations would you perform?
The patient needs close follow-up with check cystoscopy performed at approximately 3-monthly intervals. Transitional cell carcinoma of the urothelium is characterized by polychronotropism (multiple recurrences in time and space) which reflect a field change affecting the entire urothelium. The right collecting system needs to be assessed as TCC can affect the contra-lateral kidney or ureter. Either an intravenous pyelogram or retrograde pyelogram at the time of check cystoscopy are appropriate. Urine cytology will provide additional information, especially if there is carcinoma *in situ* or high grade TCC in the remaining urothelium. Carcinoma *in situ* is often only diagnosed on cytology, as it is not a raised lesion. Urine cytology from three specimens increases the detection rate.

Check cystoscopy shows several superficial recurrences which are resected completely. A right retrograde pyelogram reveals a 5-cm irregular radiolucent filling defect in the midureter with minimal proximal dilation.

What is the most likely cause of the appearance on the retrograde pyelogram?
This appearance almost certainly represents TCC of the mid-ureter. The differential diagnoses of radiolucent filling defects in the urinary tract include blood clot, radiolucent stone, air bubble, sloughed renal papilla, and, very rarely, fungal ball.

How would you confirm the diagnosis?
Use of the ureteroscope allows direct inspection of the lesion, and often biopsy can be safely performed. If the tumour has a narrow base, cautery or laser can remove the entire tumour. Non-contrast CT scan (especially spiral CT) is most useful in differentiating stone and soft tissue. Even radiolucent stones have high radiodensity on CT. The CT scan will provide useful staging information if the lesion is not a stone.

Abdominal and pelvic CT scan confirm a soft tissue mass in the ureter without evidence of spread. Chest radiograph is clear.

What are the treatment options for this patient?
Treatment options for the tumour in the mid-ureter are:

- nephroureterectomy;
- endoscopic resection;
- intra-lumen chemotherapy;
- local resection and reconstruction with a bladder flap;
- autotransplantation of the kidney so it required a shorter ureter;
- construction of ileal ureter;
- resection of the entire ureter and cystectomy followed by formation of ileal conduit onto the renal pelvis.

Neither systemic chemotherapy nor radiotherapy is suitable for treating the localized primary tumour.

Treatment options for the bladder tumour are:

- repeat cystoscopy with resection of the superficial recurrence;
- intravesical chemotherapy (bacillus Calmette–Guerin, mitomycin C, or adriamycin);
- cystectomy.

Radiotherapy is not very effective for low-grade, superficial TCC.

Which treatment would you offer this patient and why?
The treatment objectives are:

(1) tumour control (both local and systemic);
(2) preservation of renal function to avoid dialysis;
(3) bladder preservation to avoid urinary stoma.

The most common approach has been nephroureterectomy, but this carries with it inevitable total renal failure. However, a case can be made for more conservative surgical approaches. Prognosis is largely dependent on the inherent biology of the tumour rather than the extent of surgery performed. However, recurrence rates in the remaining ipsilateral upper urinary tract are as high as 40 per cent following local resection alone.

In this patient, conservative surgery is most appropriate. If the tumour base is small, endoscopic resection may be considered. However, if the tumour base is too large for endoscopic resection, ureterectomy is necessary, with urine passage reconstructed by using a bladder flap, autotransplantation, or interposition of an ileal ureter. With regard to reconstruction of a pathway for urine flow, it should be noted that after years of repeated diathermy, the bladder volume is often reduced, making it impossible for a bladder flap to reach the renal pelvis. In preparation for autotransplant, a renal angiogram should be performed to assess the urological anatomy. If variant anatomy is found (e.g. two renal arteries supplying the right kidney) autotransplantation may be more difficult or inappropriate. Interposition of an ileal ureter may thus be the treatment option that best fits the treatment objectives.

In this patient, after the entire ureter was removed, a 20-cm segment of terminal ileum was isolated and used to bridge the gap between the renal pelvis and bladder.

Are there any other specific problems which may occur?
The intestine is not designed to come in contact with urine. Various metabolic disturbances may occur depending on which segment of bowel is used in reconstruction. In the case of terminal ileum, the most important abnormality is hyperchloric acidosis. Metabolic disorders from urine absorption are more common if there is prolonged contact between urine and intestinal mucosa such as in 'neobladders'. Mucus and urinary stone formation, as well as urinary infection, are quite common. Occasionally vitamin B_{12} deficiency is seen due to poor absorption.

This patient underwent total ureterectomy with ileal ureter formation. Recovery was uneventful except for mild acidosis, which was controlled by oral sodium bicarbonate. Subsequently, several bladder recurrences have been treated by local resection and diathermy.

7.6 Ureteric obstruction in a patient with bladder cancer

A 68-year-old man with superficial transitional cell carcinoma of the bladder has been treated with intravesical bacillus Calmette–Guerin (BCG) for 4 years. He now presents to his urologist with nausea and lethargy. Blood tests reveal renal failure with a serum creatinine of 0.85 mmol/l, serum urea of 35.0 mmol/l, and serum potassium of 6.2 mmol/l.

How should this patient be managed?
The patient has severe electrolyte abnormalities making anaesthesia and retrograde cystoscopic insertion of ureteric stents hazardous. Moreover, it is often technically difficult to identify the ureteric orifice in patients with

advanced bladder cancer (or indeed prostate cancer) presenting with obstruction. A percutaneous nephrostomy(s) is the best option, this being a relatively minor procedure performed under local anaesthetic using ultrasound guidance. The kidney with the greatest normal parenchymal thickness is the preferred side. Attention to intravenous fluid and electrolyte balance is important during the postobstructive, diuretic phase. Once the patient's renal function has stabilized, it is always desirable to convert a percutaneous nephrostomy to an internal stent, either by antegrade placement of stents under radiological guidance, or via the retrograde route if electrolytes are corrected and there are no other contraindications for surgery. In future, metallic endoluminal self-expanding stents could replace the current polyurethane J stents.

Haloperidol (0.5 mg to a maximum of 3 mg/day) should assist in controlling the nausea. The percutaneous nephrostomy site can be painful, and regular analgesia may be required. Since narcotics are excreted via the urine, the half-life of administered narcotics (and other drugs) will be prolonged, and careful titration of analgesia is required initially, and as renal function improves. Such patients are prone to infection of the renal tract because of altered anatomy and the presence of a foreign body within the renal tract. Fever should be regarded as a sign of urinary sepsis until proven otherwise.

Staging of the disease is required to plan further treatment. Radiotherapy may control the local disease that has caused the obstruction. Chemotherapy may be considered if disease is more widespread, but with due consideration to drug selection and dosage in the presence of impaired renal function.

On the other hand, if the patient at presentation had been deteriorating for some time, and any procedure that overcomes the obstruction is burdensome, then a trial of corticosteroids sometimes relieves the obstruction medically, and could maintain renal function for up to a few months. A more conservative approach should be considered if life-prolonging measures are no longer appropriate.

References

7.1

Baniel, J., Foster, R.S., Einhorn, L.H. *et al.* (1995). Late relapse of clinical stage I testicular cancer. *Journal of Urology*, **154**, 1370–2.

Bokemeyer, C., Nowak, P., Haupt, A. (1997). Treatment of brain metastases in patients with testicular cancer. *Journal of Clinical Oncology*, **15**, 1449–54.

International Germ Cell Cancer Collaborative Group (1997). International germ cell consensus classification: A prognostic factor-based staging system for metastatic germ cell cancers. *Journal of Clinical Oncology*, **15**, 594–603.

Spears, W.T., Morphis, J.G., Lester, S.G. (1992). Brain metastases and testicular tumors: long-term survival. *International Journal of Radiation, Oncology, Biolology, Physics*, **22**, 17–22.

Steyerberg, E.W., Keizer, H.J., and Messemer, J.E. (1997). Residual pulmonary masses after chemotherapy for metastatic nonseminomatous germ cell tumor. Prediction of histology. ReHiT Study Group. *Cancer*, **79**, 345–55.

7.2

Meirow, D. and Schenker, J.G. (1995). Cancer and male infertility. *Human Reproduction*, **10**, 2017–2022.

Nugent, D., Meirow, D., and Brook, P.F. (1997). Transplantation in reproductive medicine: previous experience, present knowledge and future prospects. *Human Reproduction Update*, **3**, 267–280.

7.3

Scardino, P.T. (1989). Early detection of prostate cancer. *Urology Clinics of North America*, **16**, 635–55.

van den Ouden, D., Bentvelsen, F.M., Boeve, E.R *et al.* (1993). Positive margins after radical prostatectomy: correlation with local recurrence and distant progression. *British Journal of Urology*, **72**, 489–494.

7.4

Kallman, D.A., King, B.F., Hattery, R.R. *et al.* (1992). Renal vein and inferior vena cava tumor thrombus in renal cell carcinoma: CT, US, MRI and venacavography. *Journal of Computer Assisted Tomography*, **16**, 240–7.

Montie, J.E. *et al.* (1990). *Clinical management of renal cell carcinoma*. Year Book Medical Publishers.

Pritchett, T.R., Raval, J.K., Benson, R.C. *et al.* (1987). Preoperative magnetic resonance imaging of vena caval tumor thrombi: experience with 5 cases. *Journal of Urology*, **138**, 1220–222.

Ramchandani, P., Soulen, R.L., Schnall, R.I. *et al.* (1986). Impact of magnetic resonance on staging of renal carcinoma. *Urology*, **27**, 564–68.

7.5

Messinc, E. and Catalona, W. (1998). *Campbell's urology*, Vol. 3 (7th edn), p. 2390.

7.6

Chye, R.W.M. and Lickiss, J.N. (1994). Palliative care in bilateral malignant ureteric obstruction. *Annals Academy of Medicine, Singapore*, **23**, 197–203.

Norman, R.W. (1998). Genitourinary disorders. In *Oxford textbook of palliative medicine* (2nd edn) (ed. Doyle, D., Hanks, G.W.C., and MacDonald, N.). Oxford University Press.

Russo, R. (1997). Urologic emergencies. In *Cancer, principles and practice of oncology* (5th edn) (ed. DeVita, V.J., Hellman, S., and Rosenberg, S.). J.B. Lippincott Company. Philadelphia, Pennsylvania.

Gastrointestinal oncology

8.1 Analysing a family history of bowel cancer

A 30-year-old male is concerned about his strong family history of cancer. He wishes to know whether he is at increased risk of bowel cancer based on the family history. He is completely asymptomatic, but wonders whether he should have any special cancer screening. From the details given in Table 8.1 about the 30-year-old male consultant, James Reid, an accurate and detailed pedigree was constructed (Fig. 8.1, p. 109). From a review of the pedigree, if the diagnosis of cancer can be confirmed by checking medical records/cancer registry/death certificates for each of the members of the family, then there is good evidence for an inherited familial cancer syndrome, due to a germline mutation in a cancer susceptibility gene.

Which side of James' family is affected?
The cancer susceptibility gene mutation in this family seems to be inherited through the maternal lineage. The cancers in this family on the maternal side are bowel cancer (ages 28, 40, 51) and endometrial cancer (age 45). It is essential that all cancer diagnoses should be confirmed.

Which cancer family syndrome should be considered?
There is a pattern of dominantly inherited bowel (and other) cancer predisposition in this family, with four affected individuals in three generations on one side of the family. There are two major hereditary bowel cancer syndromes. The first is familial adenomatous polyposis (FAP). This syndrome is due to an inherited mutation in the *a*denomatous *p*olyposis *c*oli *APC* gene. It is characterized by the occurrence of hundreds of colonic polyps, and an almost certain risk of bowel cancer in carriers of the *APC* gene mutation. The second syndrome is the hereditary non-polyposis colorectal cancer (HNPCC). HNPCC involves an hereditary predisposition to colon cancer (often < age 50), a proclivity for the proximal colon, and an excess of synchronous or metachronous colonic cancers. Some HNPCC families have a similar risk of colon cancer but also have an increased risk of extracolonic cancers, particularly carcinoma of the uterus, ovary, small intestine, stomach, pancreas, and upper renal tract.

Which cancers feature in the syndrome?
HNPCC consists of early-onset bowel cancers, sometimes with other cancers. Criteria for HNPCC proposed by the International Collaborative

Table 8.1 Family history of consultant James Reid, age 30 years

Relative	Name	Age	Cancer	Age diagnosis	Age death	Comment
Father	Brian Reid	50	Colon	40		
Mother	Jean Reid	49		–		
Sister 1	Cassy Reid	15		–		
Sister 2	Jenny Reid	20		–		
Brother 1	Bob Reid	28	Colon	28		
Mother's mother	Lillian Brown	Deceased		–	83	Heart disease
Mother's father	Arthur Brown	Deceased	Colon	51	54	
Mother's sister 1	Jessie Sands	Deceased	Endometrium	45	46	
Mother's sister's son 1	Peter Sands	32		–	–	
Mother's sister's daughter 1	Jenny Joseph	Deceased		–	26	Motor vehicle accident
Mother's brother 1	Leonard Brown	70		–	–	No children
Father's mother	Ruby Reid	Deceased	Breast	70	75	
Father's father	Kenneth Reid	Deceased	Colon	72	72	
Father's brother 1	Bill Reid	60		–	–	
Father's sister 1	Geraldine Parker	65				

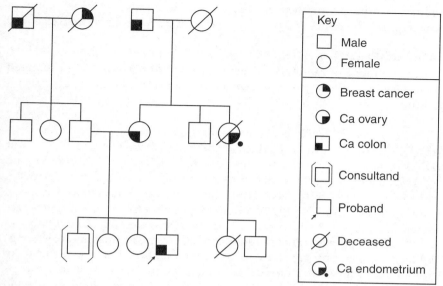

Fig. 8.1 Pedigree constructed from data in Table 8.1.

Group on Hereditary Non-Polyposis Colorectal Cancer are known as the 'Amsterdam criteria'. These criteria define HNPCC families as having:

(1) three or more relatives with histologically confirmed colorectal cancer, one of whom is the first degree relative of the other two;
(2) colorectal cancer in at least two generations; and
(3) one colorectal cancer must be diagnosed at age < 50 years.

The extracolonic cancers of the HNPCC most commonly include cancer of the endometrium. Other malignancies include transitional cell cancer of the ureter/renal pelvis, adenocarcinomas of the stomach, small intestine, pancreas, biliary tract, and ovary. The Amsterdam criteria may soon be modified to include the extra colonic features.

What is the mode of inheritance in this cancer family syndrome?
The mode of inheritance is autosomal dominant. The penetrance of the gene is estimated to be approximately 70 to 90 per cent. It is possible that up to 5 per cent of all colorectal carcinomas may be attributed to HNPCC.

If a familial cancer syndrome due to an inherited germline mutation is the correct diagnosis, what is the chance that James has inherited the gene mutation? What is the chance that his cousin, Peter Sands, has the gene mutation?
If this is HNPCC and Jean Reid is a carrier of a faulty cancer predisposition gene, then James has a 50 per cent chance of having inherited the gene

mutation from his mother. Similarly, if Jessie Sands is a gene mutation carrier, then Peter has a 50 per cent chance of carrying the defective gene.

What are the risks of bowel cancer in the carriers of this gene mutation?
The penetrance of the HNPCC genes is not 100 per cent. It is estimated that the risk of bowel cancer in gene carriers approaches 85 per cent over a lifetime.

Is genetic testing available for this syndrome?
HNPCC is now known to be due to inherited defects in one of at least four DNA mismatch repair genes. These genes, *hMLH1*, *hMSH2*, *hPMS1*, and *hPMS2*, code for enzymes which are involved in the correction of errors in the replication of DNA. DNA replication errors are found in most cancers from persons with HNPCC. Germline mutations in these genes are detectable in individuals with HNPCC. It is estimated that 1 in 200 to 1 in 2000 individuals may carry a mutation in one of the mismatch repair genes. Different mutations are seen in different families, but the majority of mutations result in the production of a truncated protein which can be detected in the analysis of mRNA from the peripheral blood of affected individuals. Once the mutation in one of these genes is defined in an affected family member, then the opportunity exists for presymptomatic genetic testing of unaffected family members. This sort of testing should only be done with genetic counselling, to ensure that each family member has the opportunity to take the test (or refuse it) and has given fully informed consent, with consideration of the implications of a positive test result, and a plan of management in the event of a positive test result. Pre- and post-test genetic counselling is critical.

Would genetic testing clarify the risks for unaffected first-degree relatives of gene mutation carriers?
Genetic testing would define those at increased risk who need increased surveillance and preventative measures. Genetic testing would also define those not at increased risk (test negative) and these family members can be saved unnecessary screening and anxiety. In addition, those without the gene mutation cannot pass it on to their children.

Carriers of a germline mutation in a bowel cancer predisposition gene are at increased risk of bowel cancer.

What are the options for screening/early detection/prevention of bowel cancer in these high risk individuals?
Confirmed carriers of mutations in the mismatch repair genes are at considerable risk of bowel cancer in the 30s, 40s, and 50s and beyond. Their options include careful screening with annual faecal occult blood testing and 2-yearly colonoscopy from age 25 or commencing 5 years prior to the

age of the earliest diagnosis of cancer in the family (whichever is first). Colonscopy is preferred, as cancers are more likely to arise in the proximal large bowel. Finally, since the risk of cancer is high, some patients will consider the option of prophylactic colectomy at an early age, especially if there are recurrent polyps with a high degree of dysplasia or a villous growth pattern. Upper gastrointestinal endoscopy is also recommended. In addition, female gene mutation carriers require specialized screening for early detection of uterine and ovarian cancer and may also consider prophylactic surgery for those organs.

In family members found not to carry the family gene mutation, what cancer screening is necessary?
Family members who are tested and found not to carry the high-risk mutation are at the population risk of bowel cancer. No special screening is necessary, despite the family history.

How does the history of bowel cancer in James' paternal grandfather influence his risk of colon cancer?
The history of a later onset, sporadic bowel cancer on the opposite side of the family has no influence on the risk of colon cancer for James.

8.2 Malignant dysphagia

A 43-year-old man complains of food 'sticking in his gullet'.

How would you assess these symptoms?
Dysphagia is the sensation of food and/or liquid being obstructed in its passage from the pharynx into the oesophagus. Features which suggest that the underlying cause of the dysphagia might be a malignancy include:

- dysphagia for solids, rather than liquids;
- consistency of symptoms, i.e. every time food greater than a certain consistency is swallowed, the sensation of obstruction occurs;
- duration of symptoms of weeks to months, rather than years;
- progression of symptoms—increasing degrees of dysphagia with foodstuffs of reducing consistency; and
- weight loss and symptoms to suggest loco regional involvement or dissemination of tumour.

How should these symptoms be investigated?
Barium swallow is the preferred initial investigation. This will site the level of obstruction and, in most cases, give a very good idea that the problem is an intrinsic malignancy of the oesophagus. Thereafter, flexible oesophagoscopy is required to confirm the diagnosis and macroscopically abnormal

looking tissue for histological examination. Two common tissue types may be found (squamous cell carcinoma and adenocarcinoma). Adeno-carcinoma is felt to be related to preceding reflux disease and Barrett's oesophagus.

Histology confirms squamous cell carcinoma of the oesophagus.

How should this be staged?
A decision needs to be made on whether the proposed treatment should be aimed at a cure if possible, or palliation only. Curative therapy involves either major surgery or major radiotherapy. Some patients will be unsuitable on the grounds of advanced age or comorbidity and staging in these patients has little reward for the patient. What is required is a direct approach to palliation.

The most widely used staging tool is high quality CT scanning of the chest and abdomen. This allows some evaluation of the lateral extent of spread of tumour into adjacent structures and mediastinal lymph nodes. It also allows assessment of possible metastasis to liver or lung. In addition, baseline haematological and biochemical screening provides information on systemic complications of the underlying disease or other unrelated disease processes.

What are the options for curative therapy?
Oesophagectomy is the gold standard by which other curative therapies are measured. This usually involves a laparotomy and right thoracotomy incision in order to encompass the involved oesophagus and a varying number of surrounding lymph nodes, as well as lymph nodes down the lesser curve of the stomach. Additionally, these incisions allow mobilization of the oesophageal substitute (usually a gastric tube), which is subsequently taken through the diaphragm and joined to the proximal oesophageal stump. More proximal lesions require an additional cervical incision to mobilize and excise the more proximal oesophagus prior to anastomosis of the proxi-mal stump to the chosen distal conduit. Oesophagectomy is associated with significant morbidity. Hospitalization is rarely less than 10 days. Postoperative mortality should be less than 5 per cent.

Traditionally, radiotherapy has been used as a method of palliation. There is some evidence that the results in terms of cure with radiotherapy might be of the same order of magnitude as the results of surgery, particularly for squamous carcinoma. There are presently a number of controlled trials investigating the role of neoadjuvant chemo–radiotherapy.

What are the options for palliative therapy?
Expandable, covered metal stents have become the treatment of choice where palliation is the sole aim of therapy. Such stents will nearly always

greatly improve the quality of swallowing. On occasions, the patient can get back to swallowing all normal foodstuffs, as long as they are well chewed. These stents can also be useful for patients who develop an oesophageal fistula. Laser therapy is now predominantly used in combination with other palliative therapies, rather than a stand alone treatment. The use of multi-disciplinary palliative teams for control of pain and other symptoms can provide valuable support.

In the context of patients presenting with malignant dysphagia, most, unfortunately, will die of their disease. The 5-year survival for patients who are offered curative therapy is still only of the order of 30 per cent. These figures need to be kept in mind, in order to give the patient perspective when offering the various therapies that are available.

8.3 Malignant colon polyp

An 82-year-old woman with a history of hypertension and mild congestive cardiac failure undergoes a colonoscopy to investigate PR bleeding. A 1.5-cm pedunculated polyp is noted in the sigmoid colon and removed with a snare. The histopathology report reads: 'There is invasive moderately differential adenocarcinoma affecting the polyp. The carcinoma invades through the muscularis mucosa into the head of the polyp. The stalk of the polyp is not involved. The diathermy margin is clear of carcinoma, with a margin of 4 mm. No lymphatic or vascular invasion is seen.'

Outline the risks and benefits of various treatment options.
The management of patients with a malignant polyp is controversial. There have been no prospective, randomized studies of colonic resection versus polypectomy for malignant polyps, and published series differ significantly in methodology and histopathological classifications.

Pathological reporting regarding malignant polyps is particularly variable and where doubt exists the clinician should review the slides with the patho-logists. The Haggitt classification is of great practical use. Pedunculated polyps with invasive carcinoma are classified into 4 levels:

- level 1—with invasion of the head only;
- level 2—with invasion of the neck;
- level 3—with invasion of the stalk;
- level 4—with invasion of the submucosa of the bowel wall.

Sessile polyps can only have level 4 invasion, as the muscularis mucosa runs straight along the bowel wall and thus invasion through the muscularis mucosa is necessarily into the submucosa of the bowel wall itself.

The two most complete series are from the Mayo Clinic. One series re-viewed the records of 151 patients with malignant polyps treated by bowel resection. The second series studied 82 patients who underwent polypectomy alone for polyps containing invasive carcinoma. There is good evidence that level 4 invasion is a poor prognostic factor, and patients with this level of invasion should undergo resection, although this management plan will, to some extent, be dependent on the patient's fitness for surgery. Patients with pedunculated polyps with invasion of the head, neck, or stalk and no unfavourable characteristics (invasion of vascular or lymphatic channels) have minimal risk of nodal spread and generally should not be advised to undergo colectomy. This is applicable to the case mentioned above. The importance of other prognostic factors such as differentiation of the tumour and resection margin is controversial.

8.4 Rectal adenocarcinoma

A 52-year-old man presents with a 2-cm rectal cancer in the lower third of the rectum situated on the anterior wall, 6 cm from the anal verge.

How is the tumour staged?
Begin with physical examination to exclude distant metastases. Digital rectal examination will provide information on the mobility of the tumour in the rectum and distance of the tumour from the anal verge. This is confirmed on rigid sigmoidoscopy at which point a biopsy must be taken for histological confirmation. Complete examination of the rectum and colon by colonoscopy should be performed prior to surgery to exclude synchronous tumours. If this is not possible due to the stenosing nature of a lesion then a colonoscopy should be performed in the perioperative period.

The depth of invasion of the tumour through the layers of the rectal wall is an important consideration. Endorectal ultrasound is used for assessment of the depth of tumour penetration into the rectal wall and adventitia. It is used with less certainty to detect nodal involvement. Endorectal ultrasound is operator dependent and this should be borne in mind when interpreting results. MRI is reliable but less readily available.

Chest radiograph and abdominal CT scan may detect metastatic disease. If metastatic disease is present, the issue of local recurrence is no longer a priority and time consuming preoperative chemotherapy and radiotherapy is not indicated.

Ultrasound suggests that the tumour is confined to the bowel wall.

Should this man have preoperative chemotherapy and radiotherapy?
Combination chemotherapy (5-fluouracil) and radiotherapy is effective in reducing both local and distant recurrence. The controversial issue is whether or not it should be given before or after surgery. No clear advantage has been demonstrated either way but the theoretical advantages of preoperative combination therapy include:

- Improved surgical access to the pelvis as a bulky tumour will shrink significantly within 6 to 8 weeks of completing the treatment, providing more room in the confined surgical space of the pelvis.
- Potentially lessened adverse effects of radiotherapy on small bowel which will be held out of the pelvis by the intact pelvic organs. Postoperative radiotherapy may be associated with higher incidence of radiotherapy complications because the small bowel can become tethered to the tumour bed after surgery.
- In theory, tumour vascularization is optimal before surgery, potentially enhancing the effects of radiotherapy and chemotherapy.

The main theoretical disadvantage of preoperative radiotherapy is that an inaccurately overstaged patient may receive unnecessary radiotherapy. The argument will continue until the result of a definitive trial is known.

What preparation does the patient require for surgery?
Major morbidity following colorectal surgery is a result of cardiac and respiratory causes and therefore these conditions need to be optimized prior to surgery.

The patient should be counselled with regard to possible complications. In the male who is sexually active, the risk of injury to autonomic nerves resulting in erectile dysfunction should be discussed, and in the female, the risk of dyspareunia should also be raised. Preoperative counselling with a stomal therapist is essential. The optimal site for position of the stoma is determined in conjunction with the stomal therapist.

The tumour must be excised with a good margin (several centimetres) of normal tissue. If this requires excision of the anal sphincter a permanent colostomy is required. Restorative surgery joining the bowel to the upper part of the anal canal is often possible. A temporary stoma may be required to ensure safe healing of the anastomosis. The stoma is usually closed at about 12 weeks

8.5 Follow-up after treatment for colonic cancer

A 67-year-old man undergoes right hemicolectomy for adenocarcinoma of the caecum. Histology shows tumour invasion through the muscle wall of the colon but no involvement of peritoneum or any surrounding structures. No lymph nodes are involved. He makes a satisfactory postoperative recovery.

What is the rationale for follow-up after treatment for cancer?
Historically, follow-up schedules evolved empirically out of a sense of curiosity, responsibility, and compassion. Since then, the role of follow-up may have been subtly altered to imply an ongoing guarantee of freedom from disease, and absence of follow-up implying negligence—the best of the 'art of medicine' making an uneasy transition to the 'science of medicine'.

Clinical follow-up is routine in most units. However, the rationale deserves close scrutiny. Most clinical recurrence occurs between follow-up visits. Arguments that follow-up is of emotional and psychological support to patients do not take into account the considerable anxiety provoked by these visits. One undoubted benefit of structured follow-up is the ability to monitor outcomes of treatment. Whilst this is of value to the physician in the long-term understanding of the disease, it may be of questionable value to the individual patient. On the other hand, intensive structured follow-up is necessary to assess treatment arms and is budgeted for in trials. Without critical evaluation of follow-up programmes there is a risk that arbitrary schedules will commit patients, physicians, and resources to an exercise which reflects confusion over the extent to which a biological process can be controlled. The legal system will continue to impose its interpretation of cause and effect on the natural history of disease. Despite this, the biological process will prevail.

Is there a role for measuring carcinoembryonic antigen (CEA) or other tumour marker?
CEA is a sensitive means of detecting recurrent colon cancer, particularly in the liver. Sensitivities of up to 90 per cent have been reported. The great majority of patients with recurrent colon cancer have incurable disease. However, some argue that the CEA remains the most effective method of detecting the very small number of patients with recurrent disease who may be cured by further surgery, for example liver resection or the occasional resectable isolated, local recurrence.

Should any routine imaging be performed?
Probably not because of the prohibitive cost of diagnosing the small number of patients with isolated liver disease or lung metastases amenable to surgical resection.

What is the role of colonoscopic surveillance?
Colonoscopic surveillance is recommended because patients previously diagnosed with colorectal cancer are at an increased risk of subsequent metachronous tumour development during their remaining lives. Regular colonoscopy, usually at intervals of 3 to 5 years, may enable benign adenomas to be removed thus reducing the risk of subsequent cancers. One must balance this with the low risk of metachronous cancer (between 1 and 2 per cent per decade of remaining life), the advanced age of many patients, and the fact that even without surveillance, many subsequent tumours will still be curable.

The complex issues surrounding the role of follow-up in both early and advanced cancer are confused and will probably remain so. Objective analyses exist to support both sides of the argument. We must ensure that what began out of a sense of compassion is not distorted by fear or defensive medicine. Recurrence can be identified early. It may not always be an advantage to do so.

8.6 Coeliac plexus block in pancreatic carcinoma

A 50-year-old man with inoperable cancer of the pancreas, has upper abdominal pain, no longer controlled by high doses of opioid analgesics. He has become somnolent and nauseated.

What can be done to improve his pain?
Neurolytic coeliac plexus block (NCPB) is a highly effective procedure for cancer pain. Partial to complete pain relief occurs in up to 90 per cent of patients. Even when the pain relief is not complete, it is usually possible to significantly reduce analgesic dosage (unless another somatic site is a significant source of pain—see Case 3.12). In addition, side-effects of high doses of systemic opioids (such as constipation and somnolence) are often significantly reduced. Adverse effects, such as orthostatic hypotension and diarrhoea, are common but usually transient and mild. Serious complications are uncommon.

In non-cancer patients, preliminary diagnostic block is usually advisable. However, patients with pancreatic cancer are often emaciated, in severe pain and unable to lie prone comfortably. Sedation and analgesia for conducting the procedure may be very challenging. In these circumstances, it may be safer and more humane to perform NCPB for pancreatic cancer without prior diagnostic block (with thorough explanation of the risks involved).

Repeat NCPB seems to be almost as effective as the initial block, unless there has been significant tumour spread. The efficacy of the procedure does not appear to be related to the radiological approach used. Other forms of upper abdominal malignancy may respond to NCPB but efficacy is less consistent than for pancreatic cancer.

Neurolytic block may also be applied in other areas such as the hypogastric plexus and the sacrococcygeal ganglion. The intrathecal route may be applicable for unilateral neuropathic pain. The use of these latter blocks is now relatively uncommon with the advent of intraspinal analgesic techniques (see Case 8.8). Critical comparisons between systemic, intraspinal, and neurolytic procedures have not been studied.

8.7 Constipation in a patient with pancreatic carcinoma

A 67-year-old male with known metastatic carcinoma of the pancreas is admitted for drainage of malignant ascites. His pain is being well controlled at home with morphine 60 mg and phenergan 12.5 mg/24 hours delivered via a syringe driver. His normal laxatives are coloxyl and senna 2 tablets twice daily supplemented with durolax suppositories and Shaw's cocktail when needed. He has not had problems with nausea and vomiting on this regimen but is extremely cachectic. His bowels have not opened for 5 days prior to admission. He complains severely about not opening his bowels.

How would you approach this problem?

Constipation in the setting of advanced abdominal malignancy is often multifactorial, with major contributions coming from the necessary opioid analgesics, together with the effects of tumour on bowel motility. With advanced malignancy involving the abdominal cavity, it is important to rule out bowel obstruction. However, in the absence of nausea and vomiting this is unlikely.

Abdominal and digital rectal examination should be performed. If the level of stool faeces cannot be felt then a plain abdominal film can be very helpful. If faeces loads the left side of the colon, rectal suppositories and/or enemas are more likely to be helpful. If the left colon is empty, then local measures are unlikely to be of use.

Every effort should be made to soften the stool and decrease transit time through the colon. Encourage oral fluid as much as is practical given the patients malaise. A combination of stool 'softeners' (e.g. coloxyl) and 'pushers' (e.g. senna or bisacodyl) should be used. If constipation remains a serious problem, simple options are limited. Prokinetic agents such as cisapride could be tried, though there is little evidence that this works. Naloxone can counteract the gut slowing effects of morphine while leaving its analgesic actions intact. Agents intended for clearing the bowel prior to colonoscopy can be used when routine oral medication fails. A neurolytic coeliac plexus block (NCPB) can make a significant difference when constipation and pain are both problems.

Chemotherapy with gemcitabine (either alone or in combination with 5-fluorouracil) has been reported to improve quality of life in patients with pancreatic cancer. The resulting pain reduction and subsequent opioid dose reduction may be useful in treating constipation.

8.8 Spinal opioids for pain relief in cancer

A 53-year-old man has severe pelvic and sacral pain from a local recurrence of rectal carcinoma. He has previously been treated with pelvic irradiation and chemotherapy. Over the last 5 days his analgesic medications have been increased substantially with little improvement in pain relief, and now he is increasingly drowsy but still in pain. He is receiving sustained release morphine (dose 600 mg/day) with subcutaneous (SC) breakthrough doses of 60 mg second hourly and regular indomethacin.

What else can be done to relieve his discomfort?

Inadequate pain relief or intolerable adverse effects from systemic opioids are primary indications for epidural or intrathecal opioid analgesia. Spinal opioids produce an analgesic effect by acting on the synapses of primary afferent nerves or nociceptors in the dorsal horns or the spinal cord. Opioid receptors are present pre- and postsynaptically, and opioids act to reduce both the release of neurotransmitters and their effect on postsynaptic receptors. The most commonly used opioid for cancer pain is morphine. Morphine has the unique pharmacokinetic property of being highly hydrophilic, leading to a slow onset of action (up to 60 to 90 min), a prolonged residence in the cerebrospinal fluid, a long duration of action, and a wide dermatomal spread of analgesia.

The epidural or intrathecal route can be used. Epidural catheters minimize the risk of meningitis but epidural space fibrosis can result in pain on injection and a reduction of analgesia. Intrathecal catheters have the advantage of increased analgesia as the opioid is delivered closer to the spinal receptors, but carries greater risk of meningitis. The infection risk may be reduced by using a totally implanted catheter system.

The catheter, made from nylon or silicone, is inserted into the appropriate space and tunnelled subcutaneously to the patient's anterior chest wall. Here the catheter is connected either to a subcutaneous port or brought out through the skin and attached to a bacterial filter. Morphine administration can be intermittent (two to four times a day) or continuous by pump infusion. The use of a pump increases cost and complexity but simplifies administration as the pump can hold enough morphine for delivery over days or even weeks. The dose conversion of morphine from the parenteral to epidural routes is usually in the ratio of 10 to 5:1. Transfer from systemic routes is gradually titrated over several days. Some systemic morphine may need to be continued to manage pain outside the dermatomal spread of the spinal analgesia, to avoid opioid withdrawal symptoms or for breakthrough analgesia.

Spinal opioid analgesia is technically complex and expensive. Additional adverse effects specific to the technique include catheter dislodgement and infection (meningitis). Pruritus, urinary retention, and the typical systemic side-effects of opioids (sedation, constipation, nausea, and vomiting) may also occur.

Contraindications to spinal opioid analgesia include abnormal haemostasis and infection at the proposed catheter insertion site.

Cancer pain may be unresponsive to spinal opioids alone. In this event other non-opioid analgesic drugs can be added including local anaesthetics and clonidine (an α-2 adrenergic agonist).

8.9 Anorexia and cachexia in advanced malignancy

A 74-year-old man with multiple liver metastases presents with a 3-month history of rapid weight loss, profound anorexia, and worsening jaundice. He is concerned about his weight loss, attributing it to his lack of appetite. He wants treatment but declines chemotherapy.

How should you manage this patient?

Given that this man is deteriorating, it is reasonable to suspend further palliative chemotherapy and focus entirely on symptom control. In view of his recent onset of jaundice, it is important to exclude a stentable lesion in the biliary tree with an ultrasound (Case 8.10). Consider other reversible causes for his anorexia and cachexia: depression/anxiety; physical causes (oral candidiasis, early satiety due to gross hepatomegaly); and uncontrolled nausea.

The cachexia and anorexia syndrome is very common in advanced cancer. It is often multifactorial in origin. The weight loss is characterized both by malnutrition (marasmus) and inadequate protein intake coupled with increased protein turnover (kwashiorkor). It appears to be mediated by cytokines, including tumour necrosis factor-α (also known as cachectin) and interleukin-1.

Blocking cytokine activity can temporarily reverse the cycle of anorexia/cachexia. Progestational agents (medroxy progesterone and progesterone acetate), glucocorticoids (prednisolone and dexamethasone), and dronabinol (tetrahydrocannabinol, a derivative of marijuana) have been shown in prospective trials to stabilize or improve weight and appetite. There appears to be a dose-response curve for progestational agents. Weight gain is predominantly adipose tissue and fluid retention. These drugs tend to have antiemetic properties as well. Weight gain probably has little relationship to quality of life and in prospective, randomized trials, cyproheptadine and hydrazine sulphate have shown no benefit in this clinical setting.

Carer concerns are a major issue at this stage of the illness. Anorexia is seen as a 'sick' state. Food has important social functions—it is the one time many people sit down and interact with each other and is often the most tangible way a partner can express their concern and love for the patient. Not eating under these circumstances takes on added significance.

In advanced disease, the question of nutritional supplements (enteral and parenteral) arises. There are no data to support the aggressive use of total parenteral nutrition in this clinical setting. There are even suggestions that patients treated with total parenteral nutrition may have a worse prognosis.

Overall, anorexia/cachexia points to advancing disease and is not reversible in the long term. It is likely that anorexia is independent of, or may follow, cachexia. This cachexia is not reversed simply by eating. The body is in a state of catabolism which can only be temporarily halted by current interventions. Explaining this to the patient and carer can be helpful. Suggesting the use of one multivitamin tablet a day is also helpful.

8.10 Malignant obstructive jaundice

A 53-year-old woman presents with painless jaundice, pruritus, dark urine, pale stools, and weight loss. Three years ago she had a sigmoid colectomy for colonic adenocarcinoma. Physical examination reveals smooth hepatomegaly, and a palpable gallbladder. CT suggests there is biliary obstruction due to bulky lymph nodes in the region of the portal hepatis.

What management would you advise?

Consider the possibility of secondary sepsis, and if this is present send off blood cultures and commence antibiotics. Coagulation status should be checked and vitamin K therapy begun to prevent coagulopathy.

Pruritus is a most distressing symptom. The obstructed biliary tree must be decompressed if possible. Endoscopic retrograde cholangio pancreatography (ERCP) with passage of a stent through the obstruction provides the best palliation in distal obstruction. Ascending cholangitis is avoided with prophylactic antibiotics. If her life expectancy is greater than 6 to 9 months operative bypass decompressing the biliary tree with a length of small bowel should be considered. This woman with metastatic colonic adenocarcinoma would be unlikely to live 6 to 9 months unless she had a good response to chemotherapy, in which case the stents may be able to be removed.

Unfortunately the ERCP is unsuccessful because the distal duct could not be cannulated.

What options remain?

ERCP is less successful for strictures above the biliary confluence (of right and left lobes of the liver). Radiographically-controlled percutaneous hepatic access to the biliary tree can be obtained and decompression achieved either through an external drain or preferably through an internal stent. On occasions a co-operative procedure by the radiologist and the endoscopist can achieve an internal stent.

The stent is placed and the patient survives for another 8 months. During this time the stent is replaced twice, using the endoscopic approach, for further obstructions (on each occasion spending only one day in hospital). She requires one admission for cholangitis. At the last endoscopy, narrowing of the right and left intrahepatic ducts and their proximal branches is noted. CT scan confirms widespread hepatic secondaries. During the last weeks of her life, the pruritis becomes intolerable again.

What non-operative options remain?

Non-operative treatments are disappointing. Cholestyramine is usually unhelpful and unpleasant to take for people who are anorexic and terminally ill. Dexamethasone occasionally is helpful. Narcotics sometimes provide relief. Ondansetron can occasionally be highly effective.

References

8.1

Lynch, H.T., Smyrk, T., and Lynch, J.F. (1996). Overview of natural history, pathology, molecular genetics and management of HNPCC. *International Journal of Cancer*, **69**, 38–43.

Rustgi, A.K. (1994). Hereditary gastrointestinal polyposis and nonpolyposis syndromes. *New England Journal of Medicine*, **331**, 25, 1694–1702.

8.3

Pollard, C.W., Nivatvongs, S., Rojanasakul, A. *et al.* (1992). The fate of patients following polypectomy alone for polyps containing invasive carcinoma. *Diseases of the Colon and Rectum*, **35**, 933–7.

Stein B.L. and Coller J.A. (1993). Management of malignant colorectal polyps. *Surgery Clinics of North America*, **73**, 47–66.

8.4

Bokey, E.L., Chapuis, P.H., Dent, O.F. *et al.* (1997). Factors affecting survival after excision of the rectum for cancer: a multivariate analysis. *Diseases of the Colon and Rectum*, **40**, 3–10.

Minsky, B.D. (1997). Adjuvant therapy for rectal cancer—a good first step. *New England Journal of Medicine*, **336**, 1016–1017.

8.5

Bruinvels, D.J., Stiggelbout, A.M., Kievit, J. *et al.* (1994). Follow-up of patients with colorectal cancer. *Annals of Surgery*, **219**, 174–182.

Follow-up strataegies in early breast cancer. http://som.flinders.edu.au/FUSA/cochrane/cochrane/general.htm

8.6

Brown D.L., Bulley C.K and Quiel E.L. (1987). NCPB for pancreatic cancer pain. *Anaesthia and Analgesia*, **66**, 869–873.

Cousins, M. J. and Bridenbaugh, P.O. (1998). *Neural blockade in clinical anaesthesia and pain management* (3rd edn). Lippincott-Raven: New York.

8.7

Polati, E., Finco, G., Gottin, L., *et al.* (1998). Prospective randomized double blind trial of neurolytic coeliac plexus block in patients with pancreatic cancer. *British Journal of Surgery*, **85**, 199–201.

8.8

Carr, D.B. and Cousins, M.J. (1998). Spinal route of analgesia: opioids and future options. In *Neural blockade in clinical anesthesia and pain management* (3rd edn) (ed. Cousins, M.J. and Bridenbaugh, P.O.). Lippincott-Raven: Philadelphia, pp. 915–1007.

8.9

Delmore, G. (1997). Assessment of nutritional status in cancer patients: widely neglected? *Supportive Care Cancer*, **5**, 376–380.

Tisdale, M.J. (1997). Cancer Cachexia: metabolic alterations and clinical manifestations. *Nutrition*, **13**, 1–7.

Gynaecological oncology

9.1 Epithelial ovarian carcinoma

A 70-year-old woman develops abdominal distension and discomfort of 6-weeks duration. Her family doctor obtains a CT scan of the abdomen and pelvis, which reveals a 10-cm mass in the right adnexum with cystic and solid components. The omentum is 'thickened', and ascites is present. Serum CA125 is 790 units/ml. A presumptive diagnosis of ovarian carcinoma is made. After ensuring fitness for anaesthesia, the patient undergoes cytoreductive surgery involving omentectomy, enbloc total abdominal hysterectomy, bilateral salpingo-oophorectomy, and re-section of the sigmoid colon. At the end of surgery, there is no macroscopic residual disease. Histopathological examination of the resected specimen reveals a serous cystadenocarcinoma of the right ovary with metastatic nodules ranging from 1 to 2 cm in size found in the left ovary, uterine serosa, omentum, and pelvic peritoneum.

What is the role of initial cytoreductive surgery in advanced ovarian cancer?
Standard management of epithelial ovarian carcinoma is laparotomy and debulking of tumour. Benefits of judicious surgical debulking (as opposed to a cytological diagnosis followed by medical therapy) include:

- establishing a firm diagnosis (excluding diagnoses such as pancreatic carcinoma or malignant mixed Mullerian tumour);
- the palliative benefit of removing a large pelvic mass/omental cake;
- a possible, small survival benefit as a result of surgical debulking improving the efficacy of subsequent chemotherapy.

Many studies document improved results in patients with minimum residual disease (i.e. <1 cm) compared to patients left with bulky disease despite surgery. However, this observation does not address the question of the relative effects of surgery versus tumour biology. It is possible that those patients whose tumours can be debulked surgically have tumours which are biologically different, and would do just as well without debulking. Reports of a beneficial effect of a repeat attempt (i.e. 'interval') debulking surgery in patients who are unable to be optimally debulked at initial surgery argue for a direct effect of surgery on prognosis. On the other hand, the observation that stage III patients who have 1 cm or less metastatic disease before debulking surgery do better than patients who have more bulky disease surgically reduced to <1 cm argues for an effect of tumour biology as well.

The extent of surgery which is appropriate in a particular case requires careful judgement. For example a patient who will be left with even one deposit more than 1 cm is unlikely to benefit from very aggressive procedures (e.g. bowel resection or splenectomy) to remove other potentially resectable deposits. An assessment of the balance between the morbidity of a prolonged debulking procedure and the likely benefits must be made intraoperatively.

Primary cytoreductive surgery remains appropriate for many patients with stage IV disease at presentation. A patient with an abdominal wall metastasis may have totally resectable disease with a relatively simple procedure. Patients with stage IV disease on the basis of positive pleural fluid cytology appear to have survival similar to those with stage III disease. On the other hand, a patient with multiple, large liver metastases should not be subjected to primary debulking. The aggression of surgery in stage IV disease should be tempered by the repeated demonstration of the poor overall survival (median around 12 to 14 months) of this group.

What is the optimal postoperative therapy for this patient?
The 'standard of care' for advanced epithelial ovarian cancer is systemic chemotherapy. There is good evidence that the drug regimens employed should include cisplatin or carboplatin. Most centres currently recommend a platinum agent (usually carboplatin) together with paclitaxel (as a 3-hour infusion), and there is good evidence that such a combination is more efficacious than platinum plus cyclophosphamide. Most centres recommend six cycles of treatment. More than six cycles leads to greater toxicity without producing a superior outcome. There is no role for cytokine support to maintain dose intensity, as modest changes (up to a doubling) in dose intensity do not appear meaningfully to effect survival. The results from studies of very high-dose chemotherapy requiring stem cell support have been disappointing.

The role of intraperitoneal chemotherapy remains controversial. A large, randomized prospective trial comparing intraperitoneal cisplatin to systemic cisplatin (where both arms received systemic cyclophosphamide), suggested that intraperitoneal therapy was more effective than systemic treatment. A counterintuitive result from this study suggested the beneficial effects of intraperitoneal treatment were seen in patients with residual disease 0.5 to 2 cm, but not for the patients with very small volume disease (<0.5 cm). Taken together with the technical difficulties in administration, most centres have chosen not to employ intraperitoneal chemotherapy as routine practice.

Whole abdominal radiotherapy (WAR) is an effective treatment for some patients. The site and bulk of residual disease and the radiotolerance of normal tissues determine the applicability of irradiation. Favourable sites include the pelvis and para-aortic nodes (where a higher dose of irradiation can be safely administered). The radiotolerance of the kidneys, and to a lesser extent the liver and small bowel, limit the effectiveness of WAR for patients with upper abdominal disease. The acute toxicity of WAR is at least as marked as that seen with modern chemotherapy, and the long term toxicity of WAR (usually manifest as chronic bowel dysfunction) is not seen after chemotherapy. For these reasons, most centres do not employ WAR as routine therapy. There is no defined role for either combined chemo–radiation or sequential therapy in epithelial ovarian cancer.

If the initial surgery for this patient had not achieved optimal debulking, what would have been the role of interval debulking surgery?

In a randomized, prospective clinical trial, patients who could not be optimally debulked at initial surgery received three cycles of chemotherapy, and were then randomized either to interval debulking or no further surgery. A survival advantage was demonstrated for patients undergoing successful debulking (medians 27 versus 19 months). However, most authorities recommend this procedure should not be used routinely in patients with suboptimal disease after primary cytoreduction because:

- such a policy would commit patients with suboptimal disease (who have an inherently poor prognosis even with modern chemotherapy) to at least two laparotomies;
- a significant number of patients will still have non-resectable disease at interval surgery, and will not be helped by this procedure.

Interval debulking should only be considered for patients where the adequacy of the initial attempt at surgery is in doubt. A confirmatory study using cisplatin and paclitaxel chemotherapy is in progress.

After six cycles of chemotherapy with carboplatin and paclitaxel, there is no clinical evidence of disease, and her CA 125 is in the normal range. Three months after completing therapy, she remains well but her CA 125 has risen to 42 units/ml. The result is checked again 3 months later, at which time the level is 124 units/ml.

How would you interpret the abnormal CA 125, and what action, if any, would you advise?

There is no rigidly defined programme of follow-up for treated patients. A commonly used approach is to review with clinical examination (including vaginal examination) and CA 125 level three monthly in the first year after treatment, four monthly in year two, then six monthly thereafter. Some authorities argue that in the absence of a survival benefit from early detection of tumour relapse, detection of asymptomatic relapse by elevation of CA 125 is unhelpful, and distressing to patients. However, in practice, most patients learn the significance of CA 125 during primary therapy, and expect it to be monitored during follow-up. An ongoing multicentre study is investigating the utility of serum CA 125 monitoring in asymptomatic patients in follow-up after primary therapy.

Serum CA 125 is a reliable marker of disease in a patient known to have elevated levels prior to initial therapy. The 'normal' level is lower in patients posthysterectomy than preoperatively, as the endometrial lining produces significant amounts of CA 125. Although a progressive elevation of CA 125 indicates recurrent disease, its broader significance depends upon the interval between completing primary treatment and recurrence. Progressive disease occurring during initial chemotherapy indicates aggressive, drug-resistant disease with a particularly poor prognosis. On the other hand, recurrence more than 12 months after primary treatment is likely (> 50 per cent) to respond again to the same chemotherapy used initially. Disease recurring in the intervening period is less likely to respond to retreatment with the same drugs.

For this patient with an asymptomatic incurable recurrence diagnosed on marker only, many authorities recommend observation without immediate treatment, avoiding toxic therapies (which are unlikely to prolong survival) until symptoms develop. However, many patients find the idea of 'doing nothing and letting the cancer grow' unacceptable. Where treatment is required, tamoxifen is a relatively non-toxic option with a low (10 per cent) but proven response rate. Other chemotherapy options include topotecan, hexamethylmelamine, etoposide, and others. Although a trial of 'second-line' chemotherapy often becomes appropriate as disease progresses, failure to respond to such therapy portends a highly drug-resistant tumour, and it is the exceptional case where continued chemotherapy with other agents leads to good palliation.

The patient is aware of the significance of the elevated CA 125, and after careful discussion of the issues wishes to have immediate treatment. She is commenced on tamoxifen 40 mg daily, but her CA 125 continues to climb, reaching 920 units/ml 2 months later. By this time she is aware of mild abdominal discomfort, and a CT scan reveals ascites, a suggestion of diffuse nodularity throughout the abdominal cavity, and a 4-cm, low-density lesion in the liver. She receives three cycles of chemotherapy with topotecan, and with each cycle has severe myelosuppression, and an admission for febrile neutropenia complicates cycle three. On review prior to cycle four she reports nausea and vomiting of 48 h duration, colicky lower abdominal pain, and constipation. On examination she looks mildly dehydrated, but otherwise remarkably well. When undressed for examination it becomes evident that her abdomen is distended. On palpating the abdomen there is a suggestion of diffuse nodularity on the anterior abdominal wall. A plane radiograph reveals multiple fluid levels in both large and small bowel, with mild distension of bowel loops.

How would you manage this case now? Would you push for a laparotomy?
The patient has a bowel obstruction due to progressive abdominal tumour. If this scenario had occurred within a few months of initial surgery, or in the

absence of known disease recurrence, the diagnosis of adhesions leading to obstruction would be an important differential and prompt surgery after a trial of conservative management (nasogastric suction and intravenous fluids) would be indicated. In this case there are factors which suggest multiple sites of disease activity within the abdomen, and hence a high likelihood (but not certainty) that multiple areas of obstruction will be present or imminent. In addition, the possibility that the obstruction is functional ileus (suggested by reduced rather than increased bowel sounds) should be considered. Although it is impossible to exclude a short-term palliative benefit from surgery, in this case and at this stage a laparotomy is probably contraindicated.

It is impossible to predict the outcome of surgical exploration with certainty. A decision to perform a laparotomy in a patient with known intraperitoneal carcinomatosis should only be taken after frank discussion of the uncertainty of benefit, and the distinct possibility that laparotomy will not provide good or lasting palliation, and may well make things worse. She must understand that a colostomy may be necessary, and, even less pleasant complications such as a faecal fistula may develop.

Having stated these reservations and noted the literature (which with the small series involved can be taken for or against the case), the surgeon is urged to consider the following (none of which are absolute):

- the well being and independence of the patient prior to the acute admission;
- the patient's expectations (e.g. how long was this 70-year-old woman with recurrence planning to live?);
- age;
- previous surgery and radiotherapy;
- interval since surgery.

It must be said that many surgeons have personal anecdotal experience where palliative laparotomy has been spectacularly successful. No apology need be made for a decision based on such immeasurable (but still valid) qualities as will to live, courage, or the wedding next month of an only daughter. Decisions made under conditions of uncertainty where protocol and survival curves provide but an illusion of control can be among the most satisfying of a professional career.

If surgery is not considered advisable, successful palliation can be obtained with aggressive hydration, percutaneous gastrostomy (to replace the uncomfortable nasogastric tube), and medications to decrease gastrointestinal secretion.

9.2 Palliation of malignant ascites

A 53-year-old woman with recurrent serous ovarian carcinoma presents with new abdominal discomfort. Over the last 3 years she has received multiple cycles of chemotherapy which initially provided good palliation, but her tumour has now become resistant to chemotherapy. On questioning, she has recently found that her skirts and trousers are too tight, she feels nauseated after small meals, has early satiety, and diminished appetite. She has also noted bilateral leg swelling and dyspnoea on exertion.

How would you assess and manage this patient?
This combination of symptoms suggests the development of large volume ascites, which can be confirmed by abdominal ultrasound. The classical findings of 'shifting dullness' are not always evident. If the discomfort of the ascites is marked, an initial paracentesis may be required. Marking of the optimum site for subsequent paracentesis during the ultrasound scan is useful to minimize unsuccessful attempts at drainage. Measurement of the patient's liver function (in particular albumin), renal function (prior to instituting diuretics), and haemoglobin (as part of assessment of her dyspnoea) are also necessary.

As this is the first episode of symptomatic ascites, and assuming there are no other chemotherapy options, a trial of diuretic therapy may be considered. Diuretic therapy is more likely to be effective if the ascites is predominantly 'central' in origin, as seen when there is invasion of the hepatic venous or lymphatic portal systems by tumour. If the ascites is 'peripheral' in origin (i.e. originating from peritoneal metastases), diuretics are less helpful. In this situation, a trial of steroid therapy such as dexamethasone 4 mg daily, may be beneficial. For central ascites, a combination of an aldosterone-blocking diuretic (e.g. spironolactone) and a loop diuretic (e.g. Frusemide) maximizes diuresis. The dose of diuretics may be progressively escalated, but the maximum useful dose of spironalactone seldom exceeds 200 mg/24 h and nausea often occurs at these dose levels. Care must be taken to avoid dehydration and renal impairment.

In many cases, there is a combination of peripheral and central ascites, which may prove resistant to both diuretics and steroids. In these patients, the only effective palliation is repeated paracentesis. Repeated drainage exacerbates protein depletion, risks introduction of infection, and extreme fluid shifts may cause hypovolemic shock syndromes, so attempting to minimize the frequency of paracentesis (e.g. use of regular analgesics, and limiting the indication for drainage to development of tense ascites) is recommended. If an appropriate frequency of drainage to maintain comfort can be established, routine admission at predetermined intervals can minimize patient discomfort and avert periods of excess discomfort. Slow drainage by placement of a cannula attached to a catheter and drainage bag, and limiting drainage to 5 l in 24 h, is well tolerated by most patients. Protein replacement may be indicated if large volume exudates are removed. There is no role for intracavitary chemotherapy, which is toxic and often painful. Likewise the use of surgically implanted drains or shunts is usually disappointing with early drain blockage or infection being common.

Associated symptoms of nausea, early satiety, anorexia, and dyspnoea may resolve at least partially with reduction in the ascites. Modification of meal size, timing, and content is usually necessary. Bowel function is often sluggish with ascites and intra-abdominal or retroperitoneal tumour, and the use of bowel stimulants such as metaclopramide and/or cisapride may be required. Patients often find the appearance of leg oedema a particularly worrying development. Most patients benefit from explanation of the cause of the oedema, and reassurance that oedema itself is not a serious development. Leg oedema often improves with leg elevation, support stockings and decrease in the ascites.

9.3 A 24-year-old woman with a germ cell tumour of the ovary

A 24-year-old woman undergoes an elective lower segment caesarean section for breech presentation at a district maternity hospital. At that procedure, a 4-cm solid, lobulated mass is found in the left ovary. The obstetric surgeon notes that the mass 'looks like brain tissue', and calls in a gynaecological oncologist for an intraoperative consultation. A wedge biopsy from the tumour shows 'dysgerminoma' on frozen section.

What is the optimal surgical management?
The majority of dysgerminomas present as stage 1 disease. The surgical procedure should define the extent of disease and remove obvious areas of tumour, whilst still aiming to preserve the potential for fertility where possible. The abdomen is explored for metastatic disease. Detailed examination of the peritoneal cavity, pelvic, and para-aortic lymph nodes, peritoneal washings, and left salpingo-oophorectomy are required. In the absence of clinically evident extraovarian spread of the tumour, a partial omentectomy, biopsy of adhesions, and retroperitoneal lymph node sampling should be performed. Since dysgerminoma is the only form of ovarian germ cell tumour with a significant incidence (10 to 15 per cent) of bilateral ovarian involvement, careful inspection and wedge biopsy of the contralateral ovary should be performed. Fertility sparing surgery (preservation of the contralateral ovary and/or uterus) should be performed to protect ovarian function and reproductive capacity. Even in the presence of metastatic disease the uterus, contralateral tube and ovary should be preserved, since advanced tumours may still be cured by subsequent chemotherapy.

What treatment, if any, should be recommended after surgery?
Assuming detailed surgical staging confirms the tumour is confined to the ovary (stage 1) the risk of relapse after surgery alone is low, with 5-year

survival rates for stage 1 pure dysgerminoma of around 95 per cent. Such patients should be monitored with regular tumour markers and periodic CT scan surveillance (say 3-monthly in the first year), with chemotherapy reserved for relapse.

For patients with more advanced dysgerminoma, chemotherapy with *b*leomycin, *e*toposide, and cis*p*latinum (BEP) is highly effective treatment. For patients whose disease is completely resected, three cycles of BEP will cure in excess of 90 per cent of cases. For patients with incompletely re-sected disease, standard therapy is four cycles of BEP, but with a somewhat higher (around 20 per cent) risk of relapse. In trials in the more common testicular cancer, attempts to reduce the toxicity of BEP (e.g. by removing bleomycin to reduce pulmonary toxicity, or substituting carboplatin for cisplatin to reduce neuropathy and emesis) led to inferior results. Success-ful pregnancy and normal ovarian function have been reported following BEP chemotherapy for dysgerminoma.

Dysgerminomas are very sensitive to irradiation, but the inevitable loss of fertility produced by pelvic irradiation means that radiotherapy is not the treatment of choice.

9.4 Endometrial carcinoma

A 62-year-old woman presents with a 3-month history of postmenopausal bleeding. Both her mother and sister died of breast cancer in their early 50s. The patient has been enrolled in a chemoprevention trial for breast cancer and has been taking study medication (either tamoxifen or placebo) for 3 years. Clinical examin-ation is unremarkable except for a slightly enlarged uterus on pelvic examination. Pelvic ultrasound demonstrates a thickened endometrium measuring 20 mm in thickness, with associated cystic change. Hysteroscopy shows a polypoid lesion occupying the uterine fundus. Endometrial biopsy shows moderately differentiated endometrioid adenocarcinoma of the endometrium. At laparotomy, total abdominal hysterectomy, bilateral salpingo-oophorectomy, and peritoneal washings are performed. On opening the uterus after removal, the tumour appears to invade to the outer half of the myometrium. Bilateral pelvic lymphadenectomy is carried out.

What are the risk factors for endometrial cancer?
Any cause of increased exposure to unopposed oestrogen increases the risk of endometrial cancer. Endogenous factors include obesity, anovulatory menstrual cycles, and oestrogen secreting tumours (such as granulosa cell tumours of the ovary). Exogenous factors include unopposed oestrogen therapy and tamoxifen. Although tamoxifen has 'antioestrogenic' effects in breast and lower genital tract tissues, it has 'oestrogenic' effects on the endometrium, bones, and serum lipid profile. Pelvic ultrasound demon-

strates thickening of the endometrium in most patients on tamoxifen. Long-term tamoxifen use, either as adjuvant therapy or in trials of chemo-prophylaxis against breast cancer, is associated with an increased (2 to 4 times) risk of endometrial cancer. Appropriate surveillance of patients on tamoxifen is a controversial area, but in the absence of postmenopausal bleeding most centres do not advocate routine investigations (e.g. ultrasound, hysteroscopy etc.).

What is the appropriate management for this case?
Appropriate multimodality therapy for endometrial cancer is a controversial area. A number of prognostic factors in endometrial cancer have been described. Tumour grade and depth of myometrial invasion are predictive for nodal metastases, hence the lymphadenectomy in this case. Many centres advocate whole pelvic irradiation if the pelvic lymph nodes are found to contain metastatic disease, but not if the nodes are negative. In the presence of adverse local tumour features (e.g. high grade, deep myometrial invasion, lymphovascular space invasion, or invasion of the cervix or isthmus) most centres would advise vault irradiation. Adjuvant radiation therapy has a clear benefit in reduction of pelvic recurrence, but has not been proven to improve overall survival. Not all centres routinely perform pelvic lymphadenectomy. There has not been a randomized, controlled trial to define the role of lymphadenectomy versus pelvic radiotherapy in improving survival.

Surgicopathological staging seeks to define the extent of the disease so that treatment can be tailored on the individual basis of risk. More studies are needed to define the role of external pelvic radiotherapy, vaginal brachytherapy, or even both therapies.

What is the role of post-treatment surveillance in patients treated for endometrial cancer?
In general, post-treatment surveillance has the following aims:

- to detect recurrences amenable to salvage therapy;
- to establish a database for audit and quality assurance within individual units;
- to reassure patients that there is no evidence of recurrent disease; or
- to manage disease recurrence or complications of treatment.

To put these aims in perspective, it must be appreciated that recurrence occurs in few patients, (15 to 20 per cent) of which only 20 per cent are salvageable. Patients whose asymptomatic recurrence has been detected by virtue of a surveillance programme do no better than those patients whose symptoms of recurrence prompt their return for review. Aggressive follow-up with regular chest radiograph, vaginal vault cytology, or CA 125 has no proven survival benefit and most clinicians recommend clinical review at decreasing intervals after therapy.

9.5 Carcinoma of the vulva

A 72-year-old woman presents with a six month history of local irritation and bleeding of the left vulva. On examination a 2-cm ulcerated lesion is seen on the vulva, with no enlargement of inguinal nodes. Incisional biopsy shows a well-differentiated squamous cell carcinoma of the vulva with maximum depth of invasion of 3 mm.

What is your plan of management?
In the management of vulval cancer, there is an increasing trend to individualize treatment. The management plan should take into account the site and size of the tumour, node status, the condition of the remainder of the vulva, the patient's age and comorbidity, and the potential effect on sexual, bladder, and bowel function. This particular patient should be treated by radical wide local excision or left hemivulvectomy and left inguinal–femoral node dissection with curative intent. At least a 1-cm margin is needed with the incision carried down to the inferior fascia of the urogenital diaphragm. The incidence of local recurrence after radical local excision is not higher than after radical vulvectomy. Radical local excision is most appropriate for lesions on the lateral or posterior aspect of the vulva. A gynaecological pathologist should review the histology of the resected specimen. In the presence of positive surgical margins, further excision should be carried out if possible.

What is the role of radiotherapy in vulval cancer?
Radiotherapy is indicated preoperatively for patients with advanced disease who would otherwise require pelvic exenteration. Postoperative irradiation of the groin and pelvic nodes is indicated in patients with two or more positive groin nodes. Radiotherapy may also be used postoperatively to prevent local recurrence in patients with involved or narrow surgical margins (< 5 mm). Some authorities advocate radiotherapy as primary therapy for patients with small primary tumours, particularly clitoral or periclitoral lesions in young and middle-aged women, in whom surgical resection would have significant psychological consequences. Combined chemoradiation (e.g. mitomycin C and/or 5-fluorouracil) can be highly effective, and should be strongly considered in patients with disease involving the anus who would otherwise require exenterative surgery.

What are the prognostic factors for vulval cancer?
The number of positive groin nodes is the single most important prognostic variable. The overall 5-year survival in operable cases is about 70 per cent.

Patients with negative lymph nodes have a 5-year survival rate of about 90 per cent, but this falls to about 50 per cent in patients with positive nodes. Other factors such as tumour ploidy and size may also carry prognostic significance.

References

9.1

Alberts, D.S., Liu, P.Y., Hannigan, E.V. *et al.* (1996). Intraperitoneal cisplatin plus intravenous cyclophosphamide versus intravenous cisplatin plus IV cyclophosphamide for stage 3 ovarian cancer. *New England Journal of Medicine*, **335**, 1950–55.

Hoskins, W.J. (1994). Epithelial ovarian carcinoma: principles of primary surgery, *Gynecologic Oncology*, **55**, S91–S96.

McGuire, W.P., Hoskins, W.J., Brady, M.F. *et al.* (1996). Cyclophosphamide and cisplatin compared with paclitaxel and cisplatin in patients with stage 3 and stage 4 ovarian cancer. *New England Journal of Medicine*, **334**, 1–6.

van der Berg, M.E., van Lent, M., Buyse, M. *et al.* (1995). The effect of debulking surgery after induction chemotherapy in the prognosis of advance epithelial ovarian cancer. *New England Journal of Medicine*, **332**, 629–634.

9.2

Gough, I.R. and Balderson, G.A. (1993). Malignant ascites. A comparison of peritoneovenous shunting and nonoperative management. *Cancer*, **71**, 2377–82.

Greenway, B., Johnson, P.J., Williams, R. (1982). Control of malignant ascites with spironolactone. *British Journal of Surgery*, **69**, 441–442.

Kao, H.W., Rakov, N.E., and Savage, E. (1985). The effect of large volume paracentesis on plasma volume—a cause of hypovolemia? *Hepatology*, **5**, 403–7.

Pockros, P.J., Esrason, K.T., Nguyen, *et al.* (1992). Mobilization of malignant ascites with diuretics is dependent on ascitic fluid characteristics. *Gastroenterology*, **103**, 1302–6.

9.3

Gershenson, D.M. (1993). Update on malignant ovarian germ tumours. *Cancer*, **71**, 1581–90.

Morrow, C.P. (1993). Gonadal stroma and germ cell ovarian tumours. In *Synopsis of gynecologic oncology* (4th edn) (ed Morrow, C.P.). Churchill Livingstone: New York, pp. 275–301.

Williams, S.I., Blessing, J.A., Hatch, K.D., *et al.* (1991). Chemotherapy of advanced dysgerminoma: trials of the Gynecologic Oncology Group. *Journal of Clinical Oncology*, **9**, 1950–5.

9.4

Morrow, C.P. (1993). Tumours of the endometrium. In *Synopsis of gynecologic oncology* (4th edn) (ed Morrow, C.P.). Churchill Livingstone: New York, pp. 169–173.

Owen, P. and Duncan, I.D. (1996). Is there any value in the long term follow up of women treated for endometrial cancer? *British Journal of Obstetrics and Gynaecology*, **103**, 710–713.

Shumsky, A. G., Stuart, G.C., Brasher, P.M. *et al.* (1994). An evaluation of routine follow up of patients treated for endometrial carcinoma. *Gynecologic Oncology*, **55**, 229–233.

9.5

Hacker, N.F. (1994). Vulval cancer. In *Practical gynecologic oncology* (2nd edn) (eds Berek, J.S. and Hacker, N.F.). Williams and Wilkins, Baltimore, Maryland, USA, pp. 403–439.

Homesley, H.D., Bundy, B.N., Sedlis, A., and Adcock, L. (1986). Radiation therapy versus pelvic node resection for carcinoma of the vulva with positive groin nodes. *Obstetrics and Gynecology*, **68**, 733.

Paediatric oncology

10.1 A 6-year-old boy with medulloblastoma

A 6-year-old boy is brought to the emergency department with a 1-week history of morning headaches, vomiting, lethargy, and ataxia. Cerebral CT and MRI scans show a posterior fossa tumour. A craniotomy is performed and all macroscopic evidence of tumour is removed. Histopathology on the resected tumour shows medullo-blastoma. A routine postoperative MRI scan however shows residual disease with an enhancing nodule extending through the Foramen of Luschke on the left side, deemed unresectable.

What should be done now?

Investigations are required to assess the extent of disease at the primary site and potential sites of disease spread. The investigation of choice is magnetic resonance imaging (MRI) of the brain and spinal cord. For lesions within the cranial cavity, MRI scans provide more anatomical detail than computed tomography. MRI scans also provide superior detail of the spinal cord and canal than the now obsolete myelograms, they are less invasive, not associated with headache due to low cerebrospinal fluid pressure, and radiological contrast reactions are eliminated. Thallium scans and positron emission tomography (PET) are being evaluated in specialized centres since these investigations may allow discrimination between active tumour and postsurgical scarring (which remains an issue for imaging based on anatomy alone).

Cerebrospinal fluid cytology should also be evaluated. The incidence of bone metastases or bone marrow infiltration by medulloblastoma at diagnosis is very uncommon, although bone scans and bone marrow aspirations are often performed.

How should this child be treated?

Making treatment decisions in oncology requires an assessment of the effectiveness, limitations, and toxicities of available treatment modalities. In paediatric oncology, the effects of therapy on growth and development, and late effects (many years after primary therapy) are of major significance.

Irradiation of the craniospinal axis will improve the chance of disease-free survival at 5 years to around 40 to 50 per cent. There is general consensus that the radiation dose should be 36 Gy to the craniospinal axis in fractions of 1.8 Gy, followed by a posterior fossa boost of 18 Gy in fractions of the same size. A further boost dose of 5.4 Gy in three fractions would then be given to the site of known residual disease (the most likely site of relapse). Using an immobilization head frame and CT scan planning, treatment can be given to a localized area from multiple angles to minimize the dose to normal structures such as the brain stem and auditory canals.

Many centres now advocate the addition of chemotherapy (active agents include 1-(2-chloroethyl)-3-cyclohexyl-1-nitrosourea i.e. CCNU, cisplatinum, vincristine, and etoposide) to treatment programs for medulloblastoma. The addition of chemotherapy to surgery and radiotherapy has been assessed in two randomized trials. Although no difference in overall disease-free survival was demonstrated in either study, subgroup analyses suggest an improvement in disease-free survival from chemotherapy for patients with more advanced disease (T stage III or IV tumours, brainstem involvement, or less than a complete resection). From these data, patients may be divided into 'low-risk' and 'high-risk' categories. In many centres, chemotherapy is now recommended for all 'high-risk' patients. Some centres advocate the use of chemotherapy in 'low-risk' patients in an attempt to reduce the radiation dose to the craniospinal axis. This may minimize spinal growth failure, the risk of panhypopituitarism, and neuropsychological sequelae. Published results from single institutions report 5-year event-free survival in the order of 70 to 80 per cent when chemotherapy is combined with craniospinal axis radiation to a dose of 18 to 25 Gy. A single arm study using 23.4 Gy and chemotherapy with CCNU, cisplatinum, and vincristine has achieved an event-free survival at 3 years of 82 per cent. An American multi-institution study sought to compare conventional 'full-dose' radiation therapy to 'lower dose' neuraxis radiation therapy combined with chemotherapy in standard risk patients. The study was abandoned due to failure by many investigators to randomize patients. Many US groups now use the lower dose of radiation therapy followed by chemotherapy in standard risk patients, with current studies addressing refinements to the chemotherapy regimens.

Current data do not allow firm conclusions as to the magnitude of benefit from chemotherapy in medulloblastoma. Improved overall survival figures may be partly attributable to improved tumour imaging with a stage migration effect, developments in neurosurgical techniques and postoperative care, and improvements in radiotherapy techniques. In an ongoing study, patients without central nervous system spread or other evidence of metastases, are randomized following surgery to immediate radiotherapy (30 Gy to the craniospinal axis with a boost to the primary tumour bed of 25 Gy), or initial chemotherapy (vincristine, carboplatin, etoposide, and cyclophosphamide) followed by identical radiotherapy.

10.2 A 10-month-old boy with neuroblastoma

A 10-month old boy presents with a subcutaneous mass overlying the right hamstring muscle. Histopathology shows neuroblastoma. Imaging reveals a right-sided adrenal tumour measuring 10 × 9 cm which does not cross the midline. Bone scan demonstrates increased tracer uptake in the zygomatic bone. MIBG (I-^{131}Metalodobenzyl guanidine) scan demonstrates uptake in the adrenal tumour, the subcutaneous mass, and diffusely through the bone marrow. Urinary catecholamines are elevated, and bone marrow aspirate demonstrates an infiltrate with neuroblastoma cells, accounting for 5 per cent of the nucleated cells in the bone marrow. Tumour DNA index is 1.33. Molecular analysis reveals no amplification of the N-*myc* proto-oncogene. Serum ferritin is 88 ng/ml.

What stage is this patient's neuroblastoma?

This patient has disseminated neuroblastoma. Since he is an infant, the prognosis is generally better than that seen in older children. The principle issue in staging is to determine whether he has stage IV or stage IVS disease. Stage IVS neuroblastoma is generally confined to infants, and requires that the primary tumour be small to moderate in size (i.e. stage I–II primary tumour), and that metastatic disease is confined to skin, bone marrow, and liver. The behaviour of IVS neuroblastoma is most unusual. Hepatomegaly may be so severe as to lead to mechanical interference with respiration requiring ventilation, surgical decompression, or urgent radiotherapy or chemotherapy. However, provided the patient survives these events, there is a very high rate of spontaneous regression of all disease, and the great majority of such patients never require chemotherapy or radiotherapy. The patient described above meets several of the criteria for stage IVS disease: the tumour does not cross the midline, and is therefore local stage II, and there are metastases to skin and bone marrow. Furthermore, the marrow infiltrate is typical of IVS disease, namely a low-level infiltrate. However, the bone scan findings in the zygomatic bone indicate that there is involvement of bone cortex. This finding precludes the diagnosis of stage IVS neuroblastoma, and thus the patient has stage IV disease.

What is meant by 'biological' staging?

The DNA index refers to the average DNA content of tumour cells, compared to normal (i.e. diploid) cells. DNA index is measured by flow cytometry using propidium iodide, a DNA stain. Thus, this patient's neuroblasts have, on average, 33 per cent more DNA in them than normal cells. Such hyperdiploidy has been found to be associated with a superior outcome in neuroblastoma compared to patients with diploid tumours.

At the level of specific genes, quantitation of N-*myc* levels is one of the most important prognostic indicators in neuroblastoma (see Case 1.1). Three scenarios should be considered here:

1. Patients with non-disseminated neuroblastoma, but with amplification of the N-*myc* proto oncogene have a poor prognosis, with outcome similar to those seen in stage IV disease.

2. Patients older than 1 year with stage IV disease and with N-*myc* amplification have a dismal prognosis. These patients have aggressive disease and a high rate of recurrence, despite initial chemoresponsiveness. However, within a group of stage IV patients older than 1 year of age at diagnosis, the *ultimate* survival rate is approximately the same in N-*myc* amplified and N-*myc* 'single copy' patients.

3. Infants with stage IVS disease do not have N-*myc* amplification. Infants with stage IV disease with N-*myc* amplification have a poor prognosis. However, in contrast to the situation with older children, infants with stage IV disease, and with no N-*myc* amplification have a good prognosis, provided they are treated. The presence or absence of N-*myc* amplification in a patient with stage IV disease is of much greater significance in an infant than in an older child.

Serum ferritin levels over 142 ng/ml at diagnosis are associated with a poor prognosis for patients with neuroblastoma.

Thus, the patient described above has stage IV disease but has favourable 'biological staging'. He is an infant and has hyperdiploidy, no N-*myc* amplification, and low serum ferritin. The prognosis is certainly much better than that seen in stage IV disease in older children, and over 75 per cent of such patients may be cured, provided they are treated.

How should this patient be treated?
This patient should receive induction chemotherapy of moderate intensity. Typical regimens include cyclophosphamide, vincristine, doxorubicin, VP-16, and sometimes cisplatinum. If the disease responds and metastatic disease is controlled, an attempt at resection of the primary tumour would ordinarily be undertaken. Interestingly, near-complete resection is often adequate, and radical or mutilating surgery is not indicated. Further chemotherapy should be given postoperatively. This patient responded well at metastatic sites but had only a minor decrease in size of the primary tumour. Following tumour resection, histopathology revealed ganglio-neuroblastoma, that is the tumour had matured, either spontaneously or under the influence of chemotherapy. Following postoperative chemo-therapy, the outlook is good, with over 85 per cent of such patients being expected to remain in remission.

10.3 A 12-year-old girl with Hodgkin's disease

A 12-year-old girl develops a cough and sore throat. The cough resolves but her general practitioner notices multiple left sided neck nodes that persist. A ches radiograph shows a bulky mediastinal mass. Excision biopsy of a neck node demonstrates nodular sclerosing Hodgkin's disease. Staging investigations at a paediatric hospital indicate that the girl has stage I I A Hodgkin's disease.

What is optimum chemotherapy?

The introduction of chemotherapy into the management of Hodgkin's disease during the 1960s resulted in improved treatment outcomes when combined with radiotherapy. A six cycle combination of mechlorethamine, vincristine, procarbazine, and prednisone (MOPP) was initially used, but the late effects of this combination include azoospermia in the majority of boys and, less commonly, infertility in girls. Around 5 per cent of patients receiving six cycles of MOPP will also go on to develop a secondary leukaemia. The combination of adriamycin, bleomycin, vinblastine, and dacarbazine (ABVD) has now been shown to be equally efficacious (in adult Hodgkin's disease). With ABVD the risk of a second haematological malignancy is reduced and infertility is uncommon. Adriamycin can cause cardiomyopathy and bleomycin can induce impairment in pulmonary function; both late effects will be exacerbated when ABVD is combined with mediastinal radiation.

A popular approach combines MOPP with ABVD (fewer cycles of each), minimizing the late effects of either combination used alone.

The British have generally used a combination of chlorambucil, vinblastine, procarbazine, and prednisolone (ChlVPP). Whilst effective, this combination again carries the risk of infertility and leukaemia.

The German–Austrian Study Group has investigated new regimens designed to minimize late effects of treatment while maintaining high survival rates. Using vincristine, procarbazine, prednisolone, and adriamycin (OPPA) or an alternating combination of OPPA with cyclophosphamide, vincristine, procarbazine, and prednisone (COPP), the risk of leukaemia and cardiomyopathy is low. The risk of infertility in male patients with this combination can be further reduced by substituting etoposide for procarbazine (OEPA).

Should radiotherapy be used on this child, and if so, how?

Prior to the introduction of chemotherapy, extended field radiotherapy would have been employed to irradiate all nodal groups above the diaphragm, as well as the spleen and para-aortic lymph nodes, to a dose in the order of 35 to 40 Gy. Survival rates of around 65 per cent were achieved. However, the late effects of this treatment would be growth impairment of the clavicles and rib cage as well as failure of breast development. Thyroid dysfunction occurred in up to 75 per cent of patients with a proportion developing thyroid carcinoma. There is now evidence of an increased incidence of breast cancer in prepubertal and adolescent girls receiving thoracic radiation. Radiation also causes late pulmonary and cardiac damage, but with modern radiotherapy techniques these problems are considerably less frequent.

Such 'late effects' were the impetus for employing chemotherapy with reduced dose radiotherapy. Investigators at Stanford have altered chemotherapy combinations and progressively reduced the dose and volume of radiation. Using three cycles of MOPP alternating with ABVD and involved field radiation to a dose of 15 Gy (with 10 Gy boost to sites of bulky disease), a 10-year survival of 96 per cent is projected for 57 patients with Hodgkin's disease of all stages. No patient has developed a second malignancy.

Several centres have omitted radiotherapy entirely in their treatment programmes for Hodgkin's disease. These programmes were initially used in countries where there were no radiotherapy facilities, or no expertise in paediatric radiotherapy. An Australian group has employed MOPP or ChlVPP alone to avoid staging laparotomies, and to eliminate growth impairment and second malignancies related to radiotherapy. This remains an area of controversy. The trade-off for avoiding radiotherapy is a greater risk of sepsis, leukaemia, and infertility.

A recently published study of the Paediatric Oncology Group is the only study which has randomized patients to receive chemotherapy alone or chemotherapy with radiotherapy for stages II B, IIIA2, IIIB, and IV Hodgkin's disease. Patients in both treatment arms received eight cycles of alternating MOPP–ABVD chemotherapy. The estimated 5-year, event-free survival and overall survival was similar in both arms.

If event-free survival and overall survival are identical for combined modality therapy and chemotherapy alone in the longer term, late effects will dictate treatment choices.

10.4 Childhood acute lymphoblastic leukaemia

A 9-year-old boy from a small country town presents with a 4-week history of lethargy and a 3-day history of dyspnoea. A chest radiograph demonstrates widening of the upper mediastinum and bilateral pleural effusions. On physical examination he has mild tachypnoea, moderate bilateral pleural effusions, and mild hepatosplenomegaly.

What is the appropriate next step?
This child has either acute lymphoblastic leukaemia (ALL) or non-Hodgkin's lymphoma with a T cell immunophenotype. A bone marrow aspirate (if there are blasts on the peripheral blood film), or an aspirate and trephine (if there are no blasts on the film), is the next most appropriate step. Care will need to be taken with any sedation used to perform the procedure since respiratory embarrassment is present in this case. Cortico-

steroids should not be given prior to the marrow aspirate, since this may result in a falsely normal aspirate. If the marrow is normal, a pleural aspirate or fine-needle aspirate of the mediastinal mass will establish a diagnosis of non-Hodgkin's lymphoma. Extensive operative resection and/or biopsy have no place in this setting.

What are necessary data at diagnosis to stratify the patient and estimate prognosis in a case of childhood ALL ?

The most important clinical features at diagnosis are the patient's age (2 to 9 years = good; 1 to 2 or >10 years = bad; <1 year = worse), peripheral blast count (<10 × 10^9/l = good; 10 to 100 = intermediate; >100 = poor), and the presence of extramedullary disease at diagnosis. The United States Paediatric Oncology Group (POG) believes T cell immunophenotype is a poor prognostic feature, but this feeling is not universal. The most important biological factors affecting prognosis are a DNA ploidy of <1.0 at diagnosis and an M3 bone marrow (more than 25 per cent blast cells as a proportion of total nucleated marrow cells) at day 7 or 14 after commencing therapy, and the presence of specific chromosomal translocations [t(12;21) = good; t (4;11) and t (9;22) = very poor]. The presence of the poor prognosis translocations generally indicate the need for allogeneic bone marrow transplant in first remission. Bone marrow activity is expressed as the percentage of blast cells as a proportion of total nucleated cells (>5 per cent blasts at 35 days denotes a high-risk patient).

Prognosis for cure in standard-risk ALL is now 70 to 80 per cent and for high-risk ALL it is 60 to 70 per cent.

This boy has high-risk ALL.

How should this boy be treated?

Children with ALL should be treated on a collaborative, multicentre trial or with best available therapy at a children's cancer treatment centre. High-risk patients often need a central venous line throughout treatment. Treatment duration is for 2 years with an intensive first 4 to 6 months and a prolonged maintenance therapy. Randomized trials attempting to reduce the duration of therapy have been uniformly unsuccessful.

What sort of central nervous system prophylaxis should he receive?

High-risk patients should receive prophylactic cranial irradiation (18 Gy), although a recent randomized trial in selected high-risk patients demonstrated that regular intrathecal therapy with cytarabine, hydrocortisone, and methotrexate is equally effective. In standard-risk patients, regular intrathecal methotrexate is sufficient to prevent central nervous system (CNS) relapse.

What are the significant late effects of therapy ?
Since 70 per cent of children with ALL will be cured of their disease, the 'cost of cure' is of significant concern. Children who receive prophylactic cranial irradiation are at risk of growth hormone deficiency and learning problems. Interestingly, other hypothalamic–pituitary functions remain intact. Long-term follow-up studies do not reveal a significant increase in the risk of second cancer in ALL patients, nor are their own children at a higher risk of congenital malformations or malignancy. Although the incidence of symptomatic anthracycline-related cardiomyopathy is low, most children who receive anthracyclines will have subclinical changes in cardiac function. Longer follow-up is required to determine whether these minor changes in cardiac function become clinically relevant.

When is remission determined and what is the value of day 7 and day 14 bone marrow aspirates, and PCR-based minimal residual disease assays?
Remission status is determined at the end of the first month of therapy (induction) on most protocols. Approximately 97 per cent of patients will be in first remission at this time. Patients with an M3 marrow (i.e. more than 25 per cent blast cells as a proportion of total nucleated marrow cells) at day 7 and/or day 14 after commencing therapy have a poorer prognosis. High-risk patients identified in this way have a better prognosis if stratified to more intensive therapy. A PCR-based minimal residual disease ('MRD') assay at the end of the first month of therapy is also a valid measure of *in vivo* chemosensitivity. While there are data to indicate MRD testing at other time points during therapy may be clinically useful as a very early indicator of relapse, this is still being evaluated in clinical trials.

During the course of chemotherapy should drug doses be adjusted up or down based on criteria other than the boy's surface area?
There is no uniform agreement on this issue, which arises during the maintenance phase (12 to 18 months) of therapy comprising cycles of oral methotrexate, mercaptopurine, prednisone, and intravenous vincristine. Most protocols will require dose reductions to be made if recurrent myelotoxicity or other severe organ toxicities are experienced on surface-area appropriate doses. A recent randomized trial indicated a slight improvement in prognosis for children with ALL whose drug doses were increased beyond surface area-calculated doses during the maintenance phase of therapy based on blood levels of the agents being used. This may be a future direction for improving survival rates.

The patient begins chemotherapy and achieves a complete remission on the day 35 bone marrow aspirate. However, after 7 months of chemotherapy blasts are again detected on a routine full blood count.

How should this boy be treated now?

The boy will require restaging with a bone marrow aspirate and lumbar puncture. In this case he is found to be in florid relapse on the bone marrow aspirate. The prognosis for relapsed ALL is determined by the duration of first remission. Patients who relapse within 18 months from diagnosis have a <20 per cent survival rate while children who relapse after 3 years have a 40–50 per cent survival rate. There is no standard therapy for reinducing remission in a child with ALL. Such patients should only be treated within the confines of a clinical trial. The standard four drug induction (vincristine, L-asparaginase, daunorubicin, and prednisone) will achieve a second remission in 70 per cent of patients.

What is the role of stem cell transplant at this point ?

There is no general agreement on this subject. Long-term studies (10 year) indicate the prognosis for children with relapsed ALL to be 20 to 30 per cent. Patients with a first remission duration of less than 3 years have a better chance of survival if treated with allogeneic stem cell transplant from an HLA-matched sibling, a mismatched family donor, an unrelated donor, or unrelated cord blood. The successful use of autologous bone marrow transplant in treating children with an isolated CNS relapse in second remission has been reported.

Fortunately, the patient's sister is a perfect 6/6 HLA match and after a second remission is achieved, allogeneic bone marrow transplant is performed. The boy is discharged from the city hospital back to the country for regular follow-ups with the local doctor and occasional trips back to the city for clinical evaluations. After 12 months he returns to the city hospital with a 3-month history of back pain, right leg pain, and a right-sided limp. On examination he has weakness of right ankle dorsiflexion, reduced sensation in the S1/2 dermatome, loss of the right ankle jerk, and down-going plantars.

How should he be managed now?

In this setting a CNS relapse is likely. An MRI scan shows several intraspinal masses in the region of the cauda equina, but no blockage to cerebrospinal fluid flow. Bone marrow examination was normal, but CNS recurrence is confirmed on lumbar puncture

Relapse of ALL within 12 months of allogeneic bone marrow transplant has a very poor prognosis and palliative therapy only would be offered in that instance. Patients who relapse more than 12 months after transplant are generally retreated and even retransplanted with different conditioning. Systemic chemotherapy is required to treat all extramedullary relapses. PCR-based minimal residual disease assays have confirmed that in all forms of extramedullary relapse there is submicroscopic bone marrow disease.

Should this boy receive further craniospinal irradiation as part of his therapy ?
The treatment of this boy's CNS disease is complex because he has already received cranial irradiation in first remission as CNS prophylaxis (18 Gy) and total body irradiation (12 Gy) as part of his bone marrow transplant conditioning in second remission. Further cranial irradiation could be given but with some cost to subsequent intellectual outcome. Triple intrathecal therapy (cytarabine, hydrocortisone, and methotrexate) in conjunction with systemic chemotherapy will achieve a second remission, but in this case whether remission can be maintained is uncertain. Not only will further cranial irradiation reduce his intellectual outcome but there is a 10 per cent risk of severe progressive leucoencephalopathy. It is decided not to recommend further craniospinal irradiation.

Should he have a second allogeneic bone marrow transplant from his sibling ?
This decision is based on whether more intensive conditioning therapy can be given, and the duration of second remission. While there is evidence indicating a graft-versus-leukaemia effect in childhood ALL, the use of donor leucocyte infusions for bone marrow relapse after transplant has met with limited success in ALL patients and considerable toxicity.

This boy has received cyclophosphamide and total body irradiation as his initial bone marrow transplant conditioning, and is thus unlikely to benefit from a further allogeneic bone marrow transplant.

The patient in fact achieves a third remission with complete clearing of the cerebro-spinal fluid blasts and a normal bone marrow aspirate. He finally returns to his home town after spending 2 months in the city receiving chemotherapy, but has become very angry over the whole concept of continuing therapy. A treatment plan is devised for the next 2 years with a strong emphasis on trying to provide as much of his therapy as possible in the small hospital in his home town. One week after returning home he develops a fever, but refuses to return for medical care for 3 days. He is eventually brought to the local hospital emergency department by his parents. His blood pressure is 70/30 mmHg, he is jaundiced, and has been anuric for 12 h. A blood culture taken at this time subsequently grew *E. coli*.

What factors determine the outcome at this stage ?
The short-term outcome will be determined by the extent and severity of multiorgan failure at the time of presentation with gram negative sepsis. More than 50 per cent of children presenting with gram negative sepsis who already have mild hypotension or tachypnoea will survive the episode. However, concurrent renal and hepatic dysfunction at presentation are particularly bad signs predictive of death due to multiorgan failure.

A much more important issue for this child and his family is the tremendous dislocation of lifestyle and poor quality of life that country families face in this disease setting. Due to the prolonged prior clinical course the family felt that they would only continue with further treatment if it could be delivered in their hometown, including management of intercurrent infections. The decision to continue therapy in a high-risk situation such as this requires consideration of what is medically possible, and what is acceptable to the patient and their family. Such major and complex decisions require extensive discussions with the family, and must include members of the treating team such as nurses, social workers, or counsellors.

10.5 Pain management in children with cancer

Editors' Note: The information provided in these cases relates to opioid prescription in the paediatric population. For a more complete discussion of the diagnosis and management of pain in adult patients with cancer see Case 3.12.

Acute pain emergency

A 3-year-old, 15 kg patient has newly diagnosed acute lymphoblastic leukaemia. He is admitted to hospital because of severe joint pain prior to commencing chemotherapy.

How will you manage this problem?
Children with acute, severe pain are often commenced on intravenous opioid and the dose titrated according to analgesia and side-effects. A starting dose of 0.1 mg/kg of morphine (or 1.5 mg in this case) is recommended. The patient should be reassessed at 30 min. If he is still in pain, but not sedated, a repeat dose of 1.5 mg, intravenous, should be given. If the child is still in pain but drowsy, 25 to 50 per cent of the starting dose (0.4 to 0.7 mg) should be given.

Once the child is relatively pain free, a continuous morphine infusion is started at 0.02 to 0.03 mg/kg per h (0.3 to 0.4 mg per h). In addition, hourly 'rescue' doses need to be provided for breakthrough pain. The 'rescue' dose is calculated as 50 to 200 per cent of the continuous hourly infusion rate (i.e. a range of 0.1 to 0.6 mg).

If repeated 'rescue' doses are required over the next 24-h period, the hourly infusion rate needs to be increased. This is calculated by reviewing the previous days total 'rescue' dose usage, calculating the average hourly 'rescue' dose and adding that to the initial infusion rate. In this case if eight 'rescues' of 0.3 mg were required in the previous 24-hour period (equivalent to 2.4 mg) an additional 0.1 mg/h is added to the basal infusion rate, that is the new infusion rate is 0.4 mg/h.

In this case the joint pain resolved following the commencement of chemotherapy and the morphine infusion was able to be stopped after a few days.

Chronic cancer pain management with morphine

A 10-year-old girl with metastatic Ewing's sarcoma is admitted to hospital with an exacerbation of long standing cancer pain. She has been receiving intravenous morphine via a PCA (patient controlled analgesia system) at a basal infusion rate of 2.5 mg/h and a bolus dose of 1 mg with a lockout interval every 30 min. Over the last 2 days she has become more comfortable. It seems timely to cease the infusion and commence oral morphine.

How do you calculate the appropriate oral dose?

Begin by calculating the total daily parenteral morphine used according to the PCA chart in the records. In this case the dose has been stable for 2 days with only three bolus doses being used in that time. This represents a total of 63 mg of intravenous morphine per day.

Next, calculate the equivalent daily oral dose requirement. Using a 3:1 oral:parenteral ratio, 63 mg of intravenous morphine should be equivalent to 189 mg/day of oral morphine. This can be administered as immediate release morphine given every 4 hours or sustained release morphine typically given every 12 hours. The equivalent oral dose would be 31 mg of immediate release morphine every 4 hours or 94 mg sustained release morphine every 12 hours. For convenience, the dose could be rounded to 30 mg and 90 mg respectively. A supply of immediate release morphine for 'rescue' dosing (e.g. 20 mg every 1 hour as needed) should be provided, whether the patient is on 4-hourly solution or sustained release morphine tablets. 'Rescue' doses are 5 to 10 per cent of the total daily opioid dose.

The dose should be subsequently adjusted according to analgesia and side-effects.

Opioid rotation

A 4-year-old, 30-kg child has commenced a continuous intravenous infusion of morphine for bone pain related to refractory leukaemia. Over the past week the dose has escalated to 5 mg morphine per hour. Further dose escalation is required to achieve adequate analgesia but opioid dose limiting toxicity (nausea) has occurred.

How can this problem be handled?

Lack of response to standard antiemetic therapy prompts consideration of opioid rotation. Opioid rotation is increasingly being used in cases of opioid dose limiting toxicity. If considering using another short-acting opioid (such as hydromorphone) standard equianalgesic tables should be consulted. According to such tables, morphine 10 mg is equivalent to hydromorphone 1.5 mg. Therefore 5 mg/h morphine is approximately equal hydromorphone 0.8 mg/h. Consequently the infusion could be switched from morphine 5 mg/h to hydromorphone 0.8 mg/h. Normally a 50 per cent reduction in the dose of the new opioid is advocated to account for incomplete cross tolerance between opioids. However, in this case, because of poor analgesia no dose reduction was made. Adequate analgesia was obtained over the next 48 hours without intolerable side-effects.

Sometimes opioid rotation involves switching from short half-life opioid to a long half-life opioid. Methadone is an example of such a drug used in this setting. The does of methadone required may be of the order of 10 to 20 per cent of the equianalgesic dose of the previously used short half-life opioid. The protocol for the dose conversion and titration of methadone has been published.

References

10.1

Goldwein, J.W., Radcliffe, J.R., Johnson, J. *et al.* (1996). Updated results of a pilot study of low dose craniospinal irradiation plus chemotherapy for children under five with cerebellar primitive neuroectodermal tumors (medulloblastoma). *International Journal of Radiation, Oncology, Biology, Physics*, **34**, 899–904.

Jenkin, D., Goddard, K., Armstrong, D. *et al.* (1990). Posterior fossa medulloblastoma in childhood: treatment results and a proposal for a new staging system. *International Journal of Radiation, Oncology, Biology, Physics*, **19**, 265–274.

10.2

Bowman, L.C., Castleberry, R.P., Cantor, A., *et al.* (1997).Genetic staging of unresectable or metastatic neuroblastoma in infants: a Pediatric Oncology Group study. *Journal of the National Cancer Institute*, **89**, 373–80.

Shimada, H., Stram, D.O., Chatten, J., Joshi, V.V. *et al.* (1995). Identification of subsets of neuroblastomas by combined histopathologic and N-myc analysis. *Journal of the National Cancer Institute*, **87**, 1470–6.

van Noesel, M.M., Hahlen, K., Hakvoort-Cammel, F.G., *et al.* (1997). Neuroblastoma 4S: a heterogenous disease with variable risk factors and treatment strategies. *Cancer*, **80**, 834–43.

10.3

Hudson, M., Greenwald, C., Thompson, E. *et al.* (1993).Efficacy and toxicity of multiagent chemotherapy and low-dose involved –field radiotherapy in children and adolescents with Hodgkin's disease. *Journal of Clinical Oncology*, **11**, 100–108.

Schellong, G. for the German–Austrian Pediatric Hodgkin's Disease Study Group. (1996).The balance between cure and late effects in childhood Hodgkin's lymphoma: the experience of the German–Austrian Study Group since 1978. *Annals of Oncology*, 7 (Suppl 4), 67–72.

Weiner, M., Leventhal, B., Brecher, M. *et al.* (1997).Randomized study of intensive MOPP-ABVD with or without low-dose total-nodal radiation therapy in the treatment of stages IIB, IIIA2, 111B, and IV Hodgkin's disease in pediatric patients: A Pediatric Oncology Group Study. *Journal of Clinical Oncology*, **15**, 2769–2779.

10.4

Evans, W.E., Relling, M.V., Rodman, J.H., *et al.* (1998). Conventional compared with individualized chemotherapy for childhood ALL. *New England Journal of Medicine*, **338**, 499–505.

Nachman, J.B., Sather, H.N., Sensel, M.G., *et al.* (1998). Augmented post-induction therapy for children with high risk ALL and a slow response to initial therapy. *New England Journal of Medicine*, **338**, 1663–1671.

Smith, M., Arthur, D., Camitta, B., *et al.* (1996). Uniform approach to risk classification and treatment assignment for children with ALL. *Journal of Clinical Oncology*, **14**, 18–24.

Wheeler, K., Richards, S., Bailey, C., *et al.* (1998).Comparison of bone marrow transplant and chemotherapy for relapsed childhood ALL: the MRC UKALLxexperience. *British Journal of Haematology*, **101**, 94–103.

10.5

Cherny, N.I. and Foley, K.M. (1996). Non opioid and opioid analgesic pharmacotherapy of cancer pain. *Hematology/Oncology Clinics of North America*, **10**, 79–102.

Inturrisi, C.E., Portenoy, R.K., Max, M.B., *et al.* (1990). Pharmacokinetic—pharmacodynamic relationships of methadone infusions in patients with cancer pain. *Clinical Pharmacology and Therapeutics*, **47**, 565–577.

Sarcoma and bone oncology

11.1 Osteogenic sarcoma

A 19-year-old male presents with a 4-month history of pain in the left leg just above the knee. The pain has been of insidious onset but appeared to develop after relatively minor trauma sustained during a football match. Initially, the pain did not interfere with his lifestyle but after 8 weeks he sought advice from a chiropractor who told him this was a muscle strain and commenced a programme of heat and massage. Over the next 6 weeks the pain became constant and unremitting. Simple analgesics and subsequently a non-steroidal anti-inflammatory drug were required for control of his symptoms. Eventually worsening pain and inability to get a good night's rest led to presentation to his local doctor. A plain radiograph of the femur demonstrates a primary bone tumour.

Osteosarcoma is the most common primary malignant bone tumour in teenagers and young adults. Most osteosarcomas occur during teenage and early adult life, before final bone maturity. A small number of osteosarcomas develop during the fifth and sixth decades and are usually associated with underlying benign bone tumours, previous irradiation, or Paget's disease.

The onset of symptoms is typically insidious and in many cases linked to a trivial injury. At first the symptoms may be confused with a minor musculoskeletal injury and it is not uncommon that the diagnosis is delayed. Symptoms which should arouse suspicion of a serious cause include pain which is unremitting and worsening. Pain persisting at rest and at night is a particularly ominous sign suggesting bone destruction/infiltration. Spectacular presentations such as pathological fracture are uncommon.

Symptoms suggestive of a bone lesion, particularly the characteristic history and examination here, are a clear indication for high quality bilateral plain radiographs.

How should this patient be managed?
The management of bone tumours should be carried out within experienced, multidisciplinary units comprising specialist orthopaedic and surgical oncologists, radiologists, pathologists, medical oncologists, and radiation oncologists. Access to specialist social work and counselling services as well as rehabilitation services is very important in the overall care of these

patients. There is now good evidence that outcome of treatment for bone tumours is superior when treatment is undertaken by experienced specialists working in a multidisciplinary team.

Staging (which should be completed prior to definitive biopsy) delineates the exact site and extent of the lesion including proximal and distal extension of the tumour. High quality anteroposterior and lateral radiographs of the affected bone including the joint above and below the lesion must be performed. Radionuclide bone scans may reveal skip lesions in the affected limb as well as skeletal metastases. Thallium scanning is useful in assessing the extent of disease and may prove valuable in follow-up and is therefore obtained as a baseline at this stage. A thoracic CT scan is required, as the most common site of metastases from osteosarcoma is the lung, with up to 20 per cent of patients having evidence of pulmonary metastases at the time of presentation.

Elevated serum alkaline phosphatase level is present in up to 50 per cent of patients, and is associated with a poorer prognosis.

An extensive tumour involves the lower femur and extends close to the joint. There is evidence of a soft tissue mass and proximal spread of tumour up the medullary cavity.

What are the issues in obtaining a tissue diagnosis?
Biopsy should be performed by the team who will be undertaking the definitive surgical management. A poorly or inexpertly performed biopsy may adversely effect the chance of limb preservation or survival. Failure to obtain a diagnosis by needle biopsy necessitates either repeat core biopsy or open biopsy. A small incision is made in a site that will be resected at the time of definitive surgery. A small drill hole is placed into the bone and again the core biopsy needle is passed in several directions to obtain a representative sample. Use of image intensification may be useful to guide the biopsy.

Core biopsy confirms the diagnosis of osteosarcoma.

How would you manage the patient now?
The addition of chemotherapy to surgery improves the survival of patients with osteosarcoma. This patient should undergo neoadjuvant chemotherapy, followed by definitive surgery, and then further postoperative adjuvant chemotherapy.

Chemotherapy for osteosarcoma has been based upon the classic 'T10 protocol' which used a preoperative combination of high dose methotrexate and vincristine. Patients in whom chemotherapy had induced 90 per cent histological tumour necrosis at the time of surgery received postoperative high dose methotrexate (HDMTX), bleomycin, cyclophosphamide, and actinomycin D (BCD). Patients whose tumours had undergone less than

90 per cent tumour necrosis had the addition of cisplatin and doxorubicin to BCD and the HDMTX was deleted. The results from the T10 protocol are reproducible across different institutions with a 5-year relapse-free survival of around 60 per cent.

Although effective, the T10 protocol is lengthy (44 weeks in total) and complex, and the relative benefit from each of the seven constituent drugs is unclear. There have been attempts to improve upon results obtained with the T10 protocol. A more intensive, preoperative protocol incorporating cisplatin, doxorubicin, and BCD in addition to HDMTX did not improve event-free survival compared to the T10 protocol. However, a randomized trial by the European Osteosarcoma Group showed that an 18-week regimen using cisplatin and doxorubicin alone was equivalent to a 44-week T10-type protocol with respect to toxicity and overall survival. Research studies underway include dose intensification with haemopoietic growth factors or high dose chemotherapy and stem cell rescue, addition of new drugs such as topotecan and ifosfamide, and the use of immunotherapy with liposome encapsulated muramyl tripeptide-phospalidyl ethanolamine.

Currently therefore, standard neoadjuvant chemotherapy for resectable non-metastatic osteosarcoma consists of a T10-like protocol or a two drug cisplatin/doxorubicin regimen.

What surgery should be performed?

The aim of surgery is to perform a complete en bloc resection of the tumour through normal tissue planes while preserving major neurovascular structures with reconstruction of a functional extremity. Limb preservation is possible in most patients with limb tumours, but in some cases primary amputation or rotationplasty may be a better alternative. In properly selected cases, limb conservation does not appear to be associated with a higher local recurrence rate (approximately 5 per cent) or impaired long-term survival. For patients undergoing limb conservation, reconstruction may involve replacement of the adjacent joint in addition to the effected long bone. Reconstructive options include metal prostheses, tissue transfer, or allograft.

What is the prognostic significance of chemotherapy-induced tumour necrosis in the resected specimen?

The tumour response to neoadjuvant chemotherapy is an important prognostic factor. Those patients who have complete or almost complete necrosis with neoadjuvant chemotherapy (variously defined as more than 90 per cent or 95 per cent necrosis) have a long-term event-free survival of more than 80 per cent. Those who have a lesser histological response have a less than 50 per cent event-free survival. The initial report of the T10 protocol suggested an improvement in event-free survival by altering postoperative chemotherapy in poor responders. However, a recent report of prolonged follow-up of a T10-type protocol did not confirm these results. The peak concentration of methotrexate correlates with histological response and dose adjustments to attain a critical peak methotrexate level have been recommended.

What follow up would you advise after completion of therapy?
Patients are followed up at 3-monthly intervals for 2 years, 6-monthly for 4 years, and then annually for a further 8 years. Evaluation of the primary site is performed with plain radiograph or CT scan. Thallium scanning may be worthwhile if a metal prosthesis has been inserted, since such prostheses reduce the sensitivity of CT scan images. Chest radiograph is alternated with CT scanning of the chest.

Fifteen months after diagnosis, CT scan demonstrated two small lesions in the right lower lobe.

The lung is the commonest site of metastatic spread from osteosarcoma, accounting for over 85 per cent of metastases. Most metastases occur soon after initial diagnosis. The prognosis is related to the extent of metastases and the ability to resect all disease. Bilateral disease is not a contra-indication to surgical ablation. Postoperative chemotherapy should probably be used after surgical resection of primary metastases. Five-year survival is approximately 30 per cent.

11.2 Soft tissue sarcoma—management of an extremity mass

A 35-year-old man presents with an enlarging mass in his thigh following a relatively trivial sporting injury 2 months previously. He is otherwise well. A firm mass is present deep in the medial aspect of his lower right thigh.

What diagnoses should be considered?
Lipomata are the most common soft tissue tumour. When they are superficial to the deep fascia the diagnosis can be made clinically with confidence. Enucleation of such lipomata is quite reasonable as long as the incision is planned with possible wider excision in mind. When a fatty tumour is located deep to the deep fascia, liposarcoma should be suspected. A number of benign conditions could be responsible for a deep soft tissue mass. Myositis ossificans can be diagnosed by the pattern of calcification on plain radiographs and if there is any uncertainty MRI demonstrates characteristic features. Other benign conditions include angiomyolipoma, atypical schwannoma, and angiomyxoma. Metastatic deposits from a variety of primary sites should be considered in the diagnosis and attention to this possibility should influence the clinical assessment.

Soft tissue sarcomas are classified according to their histological differentiation. The most common types being malignant fibrous histiocytoma (MFH), liposarcoma, fibrosarcoma, leiomyosarcoma, and synovial sarcoma. Histological subtype is not a major determinant of prognosis or treatment. The histological grade of the tumour, its size, and completeness of excision are the most significant factors determining outcome.

Clinical assessment should concentrate on excluding a primary site of possible metastatic disease, searching for evidence of dissemination (lungs, lymph nodes, and liver), and defining the local problem.

What investigations are required?

If a soft tissue sarcoma is suspected, investigations should include radiographs of the chest and the affected area. Further investigations are best co-ordinated through consultation with a specialist unit. Multiple modalities of imaging are often unnecessary, expensive, and time consuming. High quality computed tomography (CT) accurately defines the tumour and surrounding anatomy in the majority of cases. Magnetic resonance imaging (MRI) has not been shown to have benefit over CT. The aim of imaging is to define the relationship of the mass to neurovascular structures and the anatomical extent of the mass in order that treatment can be planned. Angiography may be useful in special situations. It should not be a routine part of assessment.

Biopsy is performed with the aim of obtaining adequate tissue for histopathological confirmation and tumour grading. Biopsy is best performed by the team that will perform the definitive surgery. Fine needle aspiration biopsy (FNAB) is not widely accepted because of perceived difficulties with accurate tumour grading. Preoperative tumour grading may alter management with neoadjuvant therapy considered for high-grade tumours. Core biopsy should concentrate on the periphery of the tumour where sampling of necrotic tissue is less likely. Biopsy sites must be included in the definitive specimen.

Sarcoma is confirmed.

What are the treatment options?

The mainstay of treatment is complete surgical excision with adequate margins and preservation of limb function. A margin of 2 cm is adequate. Neurovascular or bony juxtaposition will limit the clearance in many cases. Resection of large amounts of muscle can be tolerated with little residual deficit. Amputation is required in less than 5 per cent of cases. Neoadjuvant approaches (preoperative irradiation or intra-arterial chemotherapy) remain investigational.

Postoperative radiotherapy is recommended after local excision of limb sarcomas to maximize the probability of permanent local tumour control and successful limb preservation. A probable exception is the case of a low-grade (i.e. grade 1 out of 3) sarcoma excised with an adequate margin where surgical excision alone does provide high local control rates, although even here postoperative radiotherapy should be considered if surgery for local recurrence at a later time would require amputation. In all other cases of limb sarcoma, local recurrence rates after surgical resection are unacceptably high and can be reduced to a level of 10 per cent or less with adequate postoperative radiotherapy.

Postoperative adjuvant chemotherapy is of marginal benefit. A meta-analysis of updated data from individual patients (n = 1568) treated on prospective, randomized trials demonstrated small (i.e. of the order of 5 to 10 per cent) absolute benefits from anthracycline containing chemotherapy for local relapse, distant relapse, and overall recurrence-free survival. This study demonstrated a trend towards an overall survival benefit which did not reach statistical significance. There was no evidence that the effect of chemotherapy varied with differing histologies, tumour grade, or tumour location (i.e. extremity versus truncal tumours). The addition of ifosfamide to anthracycline-based adjuvant therapy is an investigational approach.

Follow-up should be planned from the outset and explained to the patient. Most recurrences will occur in the first 3 years. Early detection will make treatment easier even if no overall survival advantage can be demonstrated. Careful clinical assessment and chest radiograph should be the only routine investigations performed. Imaging of the tumour bed in the absence of symptoms is unnecessary. The results can be confusing and lead to a traumatic round of inappropriate investigations. Lymphoedema can be a problem. It should be recognized early in order that referral to a therapist can be made before irreversible changes take place in the limb.

11.3 Soft tissue sarcoma—management of a palpable abdominal mass

A 60-year-old woman has had abdominal pain for 6 months. The pain was poorly localized, gradually worsening, and associated with discomfort in the lower back. Over the last 2 months she has been constipated and noticed some abdominal distension. On examination there is a large mass in the left side of the abdomen.

What is the differential diagnosis?
The best way to analyse an abdominal mass is to consider the anatomic sites of origin and possible pathological processes. Potential sites include liver, spleen, gall bladder, stomach, pancreas, intestine, kidney, adrenal gland, para-aortic, mesenteric, or pelvic lymph nodes, ovaries, uterus, sympathetic ganglia, large arteries, and the retroperitoneal or mesenteric soft tissues. The pathological process is likely to be either inflammatory or neoplastic.

Examples of the former include paracolic and hepatic abscess, pancreatic pseudocysts, thickened and adherent loops of bowel secondary to inflammatory bowel disease, and phlegmon associated with cholecystitis or appendicitis.

Cystic lesions of the pancreas in patients without a history of pancreatitis are more often than not a cystic neoplasm of the pancreas and require a different management approach. Clinical features such as fevers, rigors, moderate to severe tenderness, and a relevant past history will strongly suggest an inflammatory process. Neoplasms cannot always be confidently excluded. In such cases, it is always best to assume that a neoplasm is present so that the definitive management of the tumour is not compromised by inappropriate interventions.

Abdominal neoplasms reaching palpable proportions are usually malignant. Clinical assessment needs to cover several areas. The mass needs to be defined in terms of location and mobility. Rectal and bimanual pelvic examination should not be omitted. Local complications of the mass such as bowel obstruction, nerve compression, or abdominal wall invasion should be sought. The possibility of an extra-abdominal primary site should be considered. Consider the skin (melanoma), lungs, breasts, prostate, and testes. Examine all lymphatic drainage areas. Systemic complications and paraneoplastic phenomena should be excluded. Phaeochromocytoma and other paraganglionomas should be excluded prior to imaging with contrast as a hypertensive crisis may be precipitated. Lymphoma may be suggested by 'B' symptoms. Hypercalcaemia may be suspected and raise suspicion of bony metastases or release of parathyroid-like hormones from a neoplasm (e.g. lung or renal cell carcinoma).

How should this patient be investigated?

High quality double-contrast computed tomography remains the most useful investigation, providing information with regard to site, size, consistency, and relationships of the mass. In addition, the liver will be screened for metastases and involvement of the urinary tract will be detected. Pelvic ultrasound may give additional information about the ovaries and uterus. A chest radiograph is important to remember, as it is the most common site of metastatic disease. Tumour markers (β-human chorionic gonadotrophin, α-fetoprotein) can be useful, but their use is directed by the clinical setting.

Further preoperative imaging is rarely useful. Magnetic resonance imaging (MRI) may demonstrate the relationship of the tumour to surrounding structures in difficult cases. Angiograms are of little benefit unless preoperative embolization is to be considered for very vascular lesions.

Fine needle aspiration cytology (FNAC) may be helpful, but the small amounts of material obtained limit the accuracy of diagnosis, and there is at least the theoretical concern that spillage of tumour cells may compromise curative surgery. FNAC should only be used when the result will alter management, such as in cases of suspected lymphoma or in cases where metastatic disease is likely. When the diagnosis is uncertain, well-planned surgical exploration and appropriate resection is indicated.

What is the optimal treatment?
In cases of suspected soft tissue tumours, complete surgical excision offers the only chance of cure. In experienced centres, the majority of retroperitoneal sarcomas can be completely excised. Unfortunately, however, 40 to 50 per cent of patients will develop local recurrence regardless of tumour grade.

Adjuvant therapy for resected retroperitoneal sarcoma remains controversial. Although postoperative radiotherapy to the tumour bed is proven to reduce the incidence of local recurrence, the difficulties of dose delivery and the potential toxicity to the gastrointestinal tract of radiotherapy must be weighed against the reduction in local recurrence offered by this modality. As the majority of recurrences, even after apparently complete resection, are local, optimization of adjuvant radiotherapy is an important area of ongoing investigation. Preoperative radiotherapy may avoid some of the gastrointestinal morbidity associated with postoperative treatment and may also facilitate surgical resection. 'Conformal radiotherapy', (in which a very tightly defined volume of tissue at risk for harbouring residual sarcoma after surgery is treated using sophisticated three-dimensional computerized treatment planning) may improve the therapeutic ratio of postoperative treatment. Intraoperative electron beam radiotherapy has also been used, but is limited by lack of wide availability.

The meta-analysis of adjuvant chemotherapy discussed in Section 11.2 did include retroperitoneal sarcomas, although absolute numbers were small. Chemotherapy is best reserved for dealing with unresectable recurrences. While sustained complete responses are uncommon, chemotherapy will often halt the progress of the disease for a significant period of time.

References

11.1
Bacci, G., Ferrari, S., Delepine, N. *et al.* (1998). Predictive factors of histologic response to primary chemotherapy in osteosarcoma of the extremity: study of 272 patients preoperatively treated with high-dose methotrexate, doxorubicin, and cisplatin. *Journal of Clinical Oncology*, **16**, 658–63.

Bramwell, V.H. (1997). The role of chemotherapy in the management of non-metastatic operable extremity osteosarcoma. *Seminars in Oncology*, **24**, 561–71.

Pitcher, M.E., Fish, S., Thomas, J.M. (1994). Management of soft tissue sarcoma. *British Journal of Surgery* **81**, 1136–1139.

Souhami, R.L., Craft, A.W., Van der Eijken, J.W. *et al.* (1997). Randomised trial of two regimens of chemotherapy in operable osteosarcoma: a study of the European Osteosarcoma Intergroup. *Lancet*, **350**, 911–7.

11.2 and 11.3

Brennan, M.F., Casper, E.S., and Harrison, L.B. (1997). Soft tissue sarcoma. In *Cancer—principles and practice of oncology* (5th edn) (eds De Vita, V.T., Hellman, S., and Rosenberg, S.A.). Lippincott-Raven.

Sarcoma Meta-analysis Collaboration. (1997). Adjuvant chemotherapy for localised resectable soft-tissue sarcoma of adults:meta-analysis of individual data. *Lancet,* **350,** 1647–54.

Head and neck and central nervous system oncology

12.1 A 42-year-old woman with a thyroid mass

A 42-year-old woman presents with a barely discernible soft lump to the right of the midline of her lower neck. Her hairdresser noticed this when her neck was extended over the basin.

How would you approach this problem?
Thyroid nodules are common. Ultrasound scanning of the general population will reveal a prevalence of up to 20 per cent, although it is a much less common clinical problem. The nodule(s) detected may be solitary or part of a multinodular process. Most thyroid nodules are asymptomatic apart from the presence of the mass.

What points should be noted on history?
Question the patient about symptoms of thyroid function abnormalities as well as progressive voice change (recurrent laryngeal nerve involvement), difficulty swallowing or breathing (oesophageal or airway compression), and facial flushing (venous obstruction). Has there been radiation exposure?

What points should be elicited on physical examination?
Assess thyroid function, the thyroid gland itself, the cervical lymph nodes, and vocal cord function. The assessment of the gland is not nearly as straightforward as has been taught, and even experienced 'thyroidologists' are frequently surprised by the imaging or operative findings.

Physical examination is normal apart from the soft swelling. What test should be done next?
The investigation of nodular thyroid disease now relies heavily on fine needle aspiration biopsy (FNAB) to detect cancer in a solitary nodule or a dominant nodule in a multinodular goitre. In the hands of an experienced cytologist, FNAB is an extremely sensitive and specific test. Not infrequently, ultrasound imaging is used as an adjunct to FNAB in the difficult-to-feel thyroid nodule.

Thyroid function tests (TFTs) are mandatory, as treatment with abnormal TFTs can be hazardous. Prior to surgery, it is imperative that patients are rendered euthyroid.

Can imaging offer anything?
Imaging, if necessary, is best done by ultrasound. Chest radiograph and CT scanning with contrast are usually not necessary except to investigate retrosternal extension or metastatic cancer. Beware of the risk of pushing someone with a large goitre into hyperfunction with the use of iodine-containing IV contrast.

Scintiscanning (nuclear medical imaging) in the investigation of straightforward thyroid nodule(s) is not necessary. The traditional teaching that separates nodules into hot or cold on the basis of scintigraphy is no longer considered important. Scintigraphy has been replaced by FNAB, with or without ultrasound.

The FNAB shows a benign pattern. What treatment is required?
Most goitres need no treatment and should be followed clinically and, if necessary, with yearly ultrasound. Surgery for thyroid nodules is indicated by the diagnosis or suspicion of compression of anatomical structures, occasionally for cosmetic reasons, and, less frequently, because of hyperthyroidism.

Thyroxine suppression of nodular thyroid disease has a very limited place. Thyroxine therapy is indicated by hypothyroidism or goitre due to Hashimoto's thyroiditis.

Radioactive iodine treatment of nodular goitre is not common, but does have a place in those unfit for surgery or those with hyperthyroidism.

12.2 What is the significance of an 'incidental' thyroid cancer?

A 34-year-old woman who reports a family history of 'thyroid cancer' presents with an asymptomatic, 2.5-cm mass in the left lobe of the thyroid. This was discovered by her family physician on ultrasound, done because of the 'family history'. The remainder of the gland was normal on ultrasound. Fine needle aspiration on the mass is reported as 'consistent with Hurthle cell neoplasm'. At operation (left hemithyroidectomy including the isthmus) the right lobe was normal. Histopathology confirms Hurthle cell adenoma, and a 3-mm focus of papillary carcinoma, both completely excised.

What further treatment should she have?
Microscopic foci of differentiated thyroid cancer, not infrequently multiple, are common in thyroid specimens removed for other pathology and in autopsy studies of those dying of non-thyroid causes. The available data

(though not from randomized studies) does not suggest that these foci necessarily progress to threaten survival. In this case, such a small tumour in a young patient with no extrathyroid extension has a greater than 95 per cent chance of long-term (35 years plus), disease-free survival. Matched pair analysis of treatment of early thyroid cancer has not shown any difference between those treated conservatively and those treated more radically. Many experts would therefore recommend no further treatment, and would follow her up clinically. Some centres would, however, recommend completion thyroidectomy and adjuvant ^{131}I therapy. With the comparative rarity of differentiated thyroid cancer, and more particularly the long lag phase (often decades) between diagnosis and adverse events, it is very unlikely that trials of one therapy versus another will be able to be conducted.

Are thyroid cancers familial?
Thyroid cancers arise from follicular cells or the parafollicular (c) cells. Some medullary cancers from the parafollicular cells carry a mutation that may be familial or may have arisen spontaneously (see Case 1.2). These tumours may be isolated or be part of a syndrome—multiple endocrine neoplasia (MEN) type 2. In contrast, differentiated thyroid cancers with origin from the follicular cells have not been shown to harbour germ line mutations and have no apparent familial predisposition. In this case there would be doubt about the patients report of a 'family history' of thyroid cancer. Details of how to take and construct a family cancer history are described in Cases 3.1 and 8.1.

Does the Hurthle cell histology have any particular implications?
Although all Hurthle cell neoplasms were once considered potentially malignant, it is now accepted that a Hurthle cell adenoma is a histological variant of follicular adenoma. Thus the Hurthle cell morphology is a pathological curiosity, without other implications.

12.3 A 56-year-old man presents with a cervical mass

A 56-year-old man presents with a 1.5-cm painless mass in the midcervical region. He has been a heavy smoker for many years.

What are the diagnostic possibilities?
Any neck mass in the older age group is by definition suspicious, but occasionally benign masses such as branchial cysts do occur. Make a benign diagnosis with great caution in the over 50 age group.

The commonest primary site for metastatic neck nodes is the upper aerodigestive tract—the mouth, pharynx (naso-, oro-, or hypo-), and larynx.

These are almost always squamous carcinoma (HNSCC), and mostly related to long-term smoking and drinking. The next most common primary site is skin. Squamous carcinomas are most frequent, but melanoma, Merkel cell, and, rarely, adnexal carcinomas are also seen. Thyroid and salivary carcinoma present with palpable metastases less frequently. The only known aetiological factor for these tumours is exposure to ionizing radiation. These tumours are more typically seen in a younger population than squamous cell carcinomas (melanoma is an exception).

The position of the mass gives the experienced clinician an indication of its origin. Only masses immediately above the clavicle (level IV and V) are likely to originate below the clavicle. Lymphoscintigraphy performed during sentinel node biopsy has recently demonstrated that the anticipated lymphatic pathways are not nearly as predictable as has been thought, and thus accepted patterns of spread are indications only.

In HNSCC, those masses in the submandibular triangle (level 1) most commonly arise from the oral cavity, those at the level of the high deep cervical (level II) or mid deep cervical (level III), from the pharynx or larynx. Lower deep cervical (level IV) are uncommon, and generally arise from the hypopharynx. Level V (posterior triangle) nodes are very uncommon except where there is gross nodal involvement at other levels. Nasopharyngeal cancer (NPC) is the exception to this rule, commonly metastasising to the accessory chain of nodes. Multiple levels are not uncommonly involved and spread to other levels can be antegrade or retrograde from the original node or can occur synchronously.

Intraparotid lymph node metastases are seen most frequently from skin cancers, but almost never from another site. Level I, II, and upper V are also frequently involved with skin metastases. Thyroid cancer metastases are seen at every level except I. Bilateral metastases are indicative of lesions near the midline, or multiple primaries with lesion(s) on each side of the midline.

How is physical examination performed?
Physical examination is a skill requiring special instrumentation, in particular directed lighting, a mirror, and often office endoscopy. The skin of the face and scalp is examined in a good light. Do not forget the external auditory meatus. Remove dentures and examine the tongue, floor of mouth, palate, and buccal mucosa. Have the patient poke out their tongue (looking for asymmetry) and use bimanual palpation. Examine the parotid, other salivary glands, and the thyroid.

How would a precise diagnosis of the neck lump be made?
Fine needle aspiration biopsy (FNAB) is the cornerstone of diagnosis for malignant neck lumps, and the requirement for open biopsy is minimal except for lymphoma.

What if the office-based physical examination is normal?
Examination under anaesthetic, including direct laryngoscopy and oeso-phagoscopy, is integral to the complete physical assessment where HNSCC is suspected.

In this man's case, a 10-mm ulcer is found in the hypopharynx and biopsy shows squamous cell carcinoma which confirms the FNAB cytology.

Should imaging be obtained?
Imaging of the neck is required when malignancy is suspected. Contrast CT is the current modality of choice; the place of MRI in this context is as yet not well defined. Contrast CT is significantly more sensitive than physical examination in detecting nodal metastases. Ultrasound, except as an adjunct to FNA, has very limited use in the neck although it is the best modality for imaging the thyroid gland. In most epithelial cancers, chest radiograph is the only useful staging for distant disease. In HNSCC, there is a small incidence of synchronous primary lung cancers, because of the common aetiological agents. Chest radiograph is more sensitive and has largely supplanted bronchoscopy as a routine in these patients.

How is treatment planned?
Treatment should be planned in a multidisciplinary setting with input from surgeons, radiation and medical oncologists, and palliative care physicians. Head and neck tumours, or their treatment, may significantly impact on the ability to speak and swallow and it is imperative that involvement of nutritionists and speech therapists be considered. Dental assessment of any patient who will receive radiation to the jaw is likewise essential as the treatment of dental sepsis after radiation can lead to the disastrous complication of osteoradionecrosis.

12.4 A pain emergency in a patient with head and neck cancer

A 46-year-old man with cancer of the tongue has had multiple resections and recurrences in the tongue and posterior pharynx, the last of which required grafting. He has needed increasing amounts of morphine to control his pain which is mainly experienced in the side of the neck and head. He has been taking 600 mg of sustained release morphine per day. He presents now to the emergency department with an dramatic increase in pain over the past 3 days. He has been given an extra 125 mg of morphine by subcutaneous bolus injections since arriving in the emergency department 6 hours ago, but is still complaining of excruciating pain. He can barely talk but is able to say that he rates the pain '25 out of 10' in intensity and that he wants a lethal injection if nothing can be done to relieve the pain.

What can be done in this situation?

This patient is having an acute, overwhelmingly severe exacerbation of his long-standing chronic cancer pain. The cancer pain literature refers to such events as 'breakthrough pain' but in this case it should rightfully be called a 'cancer pain emergency'.

The patient needs a comprehensive assessment of the pain, treatment of the underlying cause if possible, and optimization of his analgesic regimen. The latter step involves increasing the regularly scheduled opioid, considering the addition of coanalgesics, and increased use of breakthrough doses.

The pharmacokinetics and pharmacodynamics of breakthrough analgesics has not been studied. A drug with a short half-life and rapid onset of action is recommended on empirical grounds. In the case of patients on morphine, such as this patient, a short acting morphine preparation by the same route (e.g. morphine mixture if he is already taking sustained release preparations) is used. There are no uniform recommendations for how much should be given, but the standard rescue dose reflects the baseline chronic dose. Some clinicians use 5 to 10 per cent of the total daily dose administered every 2 to 3 h as needed. An alternate approach, giving 100 per cent of the regular 4-hourly dose, has been recommended. In the case of predictable incident pain, a rescue dose taken 30 to 60 min before activity can prevent breakthrough pain.

Occasional patients on oral morphine find supplementary oral doses too slow in onset or ineffective. Parenteral administration of an opioid should be considered in such cases. The recent advent of PCA ('*patient controlled analgesia*') systems for ambulatory patients can expedite the administration of supplemental doses, allowing an adequate level of analgesia to be obtained rapidly.

In this patient's case, PCA intravenous morphine was commenced at an initial basal rate of 5 mg/h and boluses of 5 mg with no lock out period. This regimen was reviewed after 12 h and, based on his PCA usage, the dose increased to 20 mg/h and the bolus to 20 mg. By this time he was much more comfortable and rated his pain 5 out of 10, and showed no evidence of morphine toxicity. The dose was maintained over the next 36 h, by which time he had become pain free. At this stage he was receiving the equivalent of 4.2 g of oral morphine per day. The dose was gradually reduced over the next 5 days to the equivalent of 1600 mg of oral morphine. He was discharged a week later with good pain relief on this dose of sustained release oral morphine.

12.5 Primary brain tumour

A 54-year-old man presents to his family doctor with a 3-month history of frontal headache, worse on awakening. His wife describes an alteration in his personality, with increased forgetfulness, an indifference to his state of dress and hygiene, and emotional lability. Neurological examination reveals no focal neurological signs but you note a lack of insight with associated poor abstract thought. There is bilateral papilloedema. CT scan of the brain reveals a large enhancing right frontal lobe mass.

What is the differential diagnosis?
An enhancing brain lesion in this age group will fall into one of the following categories:

Non-neoplastic lesions:
- cerebral abscess
- resolving cerebral infarct
- giant aneurysm
- arteriovenous malformation
- cerebral contusion
- radiation necrosis.

Neoplastic lesions:
- primary brain tumours
  glioma
  astrocytoma
  meningioma
  lymphoma
- secondary brain tumours
  renal cell, lung, malignant melanoma, bowel, and breast cancer.

Given the history, glioma (particularly the grade IV subtype glioblastoma multiforme, or GBM) is the most likely diagnosis. A tissue diagnosis is the ultimate diagnostic requirement (see Cases 2.1 and 2.3).

What management would you recommend?
The patient should be commenced on dexamethasone, typically 8 mg initially followed by 4 mg 4 times a day to reduce vasogenic oedema associated with the tumour. Remember the potential for induction or exacerbation of diabetes from steroids, and also prescribe prophylactic oral nystatin mouthwash.

Cytoreductive surgery to reduce mass effect will prolong survival, but is only practical if the tumour is well defined radiologically and in a non-eloquent region of the brain. Decompression is preferable to biopsy alone. Since tumour cells are often present in the oedematous region surrounding the region of enhancement, total tumour resection is seldom possible. Cytoreductive surgery should be followed by external beam radiation (4000 cGy whole-brain plus 1500 to 2000 cGy to the tumour bed). Although this approach does not provide cure, it clearly prolongs quality survival.

Most gliomas recur at the site of primary disease. Although repeat surgical debulking extends survival, the morbidity is much higher than for the initial operation with a three-fold increase in infection rate, and an increase in wound dehiscence, particularly after radiotherapy.

What is his prognosis?

Assuming a protocol of surgical resection, followed cranial irradiation, the 1-year survival rate is only 35 per cent with an 8 to 12 per cent of patients alive at 2 years.

12.6 Intramedullary spinal cord tumours

A 42-year-old man presents with a 5-year history of increasing clumsiness of gait and 3 to 6 months of altered bladder sensation and urinary incontinence. He also notes vague mid-thoracic back pain which wakes him at night and is worse on lying down. Physical examination reveals mild diffuse lower limb weakness, flexor plantar reflexes, and decreased pinprick sensation on the right side below T8. No sphincteric change is noted. MRI of the spine reveals diffuse expansion of the cord between T3 and T8 with an associated cystic component. Enhancement with gadolinium is present.

What diagnoses would you consider?

This case illustrates the typical presentation of an intramedullary spinal cord tumour. Pain (local back pain, radicular pain, or non-dermatomal dysaesthetic burning pain) is the most common feature. Pain on lying down is classical. Typical features in this case include age of onset (3rd to 5th decade) and the presence of symptoms for months or years.

Most are astrocytomas or ependymomas. Rarer causes include glioblastoma multiforme, dermoid tumour, haemangioblastoma, oligodendroglioma, teratomata, and cavernous haemangioma.

Children commonly present with a gait disorder secondary to long tract involvement and may even have a syringomyelia-like presentation. Dissociated sensory loss is common and parethesia in a radicular or medullary distribution may occur. Bladder dysfunction is more common than bowel sphincter changes. Impotence may occur.

What treatment should be offered?

Total resection is preferred but the lack of a clear cleavage plain and the risk of worsening neurological deficit usually temper this objective. With astrocytomas, radical removal is rarely possible, and the long-term functional results are worse than those for ependymoma. Recurrence rate over 4 to 5 years is 50 per cent. Radiotherapy has a role for high grade lesions.

References

12.3

Million, R. and Cassisi, N. (1994). The *management of head and neck cancer* (2nd edn). Lippincott: Philadelphia.

12.4

Hanks, G.W., Portenoy, R.K., MacDonald, N., and O'Neill, W.M. (1993). Difficult pain problems. In *Oxford text book of palliative medicine* (ed Doyle, D., Hanks, G.W.C., and McDonald, N.) pp. 257–274. Oxford University Press.

Portenoy, R.K. and Hagen, N.A. (1990). Breakthrough pain: definition, prevalence and characteristics. *Pain*, **41**, 273–81.

12.5

Kaye, A.K. and Laws, E.R. Jr (1995). *Brain tumors. An encyclopedic approach.* Churchill Livingstone: Melbourne.

12.6

Hirano, A. (1997). Neuropathology of tumours of the spinal cord: the Montefiore experience. *Brain Tumor Pathology*, **14**, 1–4.

McCormick, P.C. and Stein, B.M. (1990). Intramedullary tumors in adults. *Neurosurgery Clinics of North America*, **1**, 609–630.

Newton, H.B., Newton, C.L., Gatens, C., Hebert, R., and Pack, R. (1995). Spinal cord tumors: review of etiology, diagnosis, and multidisciplinary approach to treatment. *Cancer Practice*, **3**, 207–18.

Managing the end of life

13.1 Breaking bad news

You are asked to see a 73-year-old man who was treated 5 years ago with radical pelvic irradiation for prostate cancer. A short time later he developed bone metastases which have become refractory to hormonal treatment. His main problem is back pain, worse on movement, despite recent palliative radiotherapy to his thoracic spine. He has had further radiotherapy to his pelvis for perineal pain due to local progression. He has just received a third course of chemotherapy from which he is obtaining little benefit. His other complaints are lack of energy, poor appetite, constipation, and weight loss. He takes a sustained release morphine preparation and some paracetamol, and is not very satisfied with his pain control or his life in general. He comes to the Outpatient Clinic with his wife. His disease is advanced and progressing quickly and his prognosis is limited. You feel the time has come to refer him on to the Palliative Care Service for continuing care. How will you break this to him?

Informing someone that they have a serious disease, whether it be a diagnosis of cancer, recurrent disease, or that he/she has reached the terminal stage is a communication task which challenges all clinicians. Whilst much is written on this topic, the majority of articles present anecdotal expert opinion. However, a number of evidence-based and consensus-based guidelines on breaking bad news have recently been developed, such as that produced by the New South Wales Cancer Council.

Models of best practice have varied across time and place. In Western societies, non-disclosure was widely favoured in earlier decades. This model assumes that sickness makes the patient incompetent, and therefore places the responsibility for deciding what constitutes benefit or harm firmly upon the doctor. According to this model, providing information which portrays a gloomy prognosis or offering choice in treatments may cause psychological distress in some patients, albeit temporary; therefore it is advisable to 'first, do no harm' and withhold information. In countries such as Japan, a large percentage of doctors still hold the view that non-disclosure best serves the needs of patients and families.

With the shift in medical ethics towards principles of autonomy rather than paternalism, and to some extent influenced by medico-legal concerns, the popular approach in most Western societies changed to one of full disclosure. This model recognizes the need to respect the patient's integrity and right to self-determination. It assumes that the patient wants information and involvement in decision making and is competent to assume this role. Indeed, in most countries, there is now a legal requirement to provide the basic information required for informed consent to all patients.

Today, individualized disclosure is the favoured approach. This involves tailoring the amount and rate of information provided to the desires of the individual patient, through a process of open negotiation. In effect, though perhaps not in these specific words, one is saying: 'Some patients like to be told what is likely to happen in the future; others like to deal with each day as it comes. What would you prefer?'

Survey data suggests that the majority of patients, in most cultures, prefer to be told their diagnosis, their chances of cure, the treatment options, and the odds of treatment achieving its goals. However, in almost all studies, a minority state a preference for minimal information. These patients may cope with adversity by screening out negative information, focusing on day-to-day activities, and allowing others to make the necessary decisions about their care. At the time of diagnosis or recurrence when patients are feeling particularly vulnerable, some patients may be likely to adopt such a coping style. There is some evidence that as time goes by and the situation becomes less acute, such patients shift towards seeking more information and involvement in treatment decisions. It is for this reason that current guidelines emphasize the importance of continuously negotiating with patients about the amount and type of information they want, and remaining sensitive to the patient's capacity to take new information.

It is well documented that patients fail to take in much of what they are told in a breaking bad news consultation, either because they are in shock or because the information is unfamiliar, jargonistic, or poorly presented. For example 142 patients attending an initial consultation with one oncologist remembered 1 week, later on average, 25 per cent of the points covered and 45 per cent of the six points nominated as crucial by the oncologist.

Continued misunderstanding of important information is not uncommon. For example in one series of 100 cancer patients surveyed, 33 per cent with metastatic disease in fact believed their disease was localized, 34 per cent being treated palliatively believed that their treatment would lead to cure, and 10 per cent being treated for cure believed they were being treated palliatively. Yet all of the doctors concerned believed they had given the correct information in the consultation. This documented poor recall in patients receiving bad news suggests it is prudent to check their understanding at every stage. Depending on the patient's current level of understanding, different amounts and types of information may need to be provided. It is important to avoid jargon, present information simply and in a clear sequence, and encourage the patient to ask questions. An audiotape of the consultation, written materials, and visual aids and an opportunity to review the information with another health professional such as a nurse, may also assist patients to take in important information.

Emotional reactions to bad news vary, but common responses include shock, anger, denial, sadness, a determination to defeat the disease, acceptance, and despair. These responses may all occur in the same individual at different times along the time course of the disease. In recognition of the emotional impact of bad news, a range of practical arrangements and interactional skills are recommended to optimize the outcome. These include ensuring privacy and adequate time, acknowledging and legitimizing feelings, offering assistance to help others, providing information about support services, and providing phone numbers and names of people who can answer questions at any time. It is also important to emphasize the hopeful aspects of the situation, whether it be the probability of cure, the likelihood that treatment will extend life, the existence of long-term survivors, or the ability to control symptoms and maintain a good quality of life. A number of studies have documented patients' desire for such hopeful communication, and the benefits it has on long-term psychological adjustment and even survival.

While the strategies described above can be helpful, breaking bad news is always a sad experience. It is important for health professionals to acknowledge their feelings at the end of such a consultation and to find constructive ways of debriefing, such as talking to colleagues, identifying what went well in the consultation, or deliberately relaxing.

13.2 'Be honest doctor, how long have I got?'

The patient looks you in the eye and says, 'Be honest doctor, how long have I got?'

How do respond to this question?
This is one of the common yet most difficult problems facing doctors caring for patients with cancer. One inadequate approach would be to say:

'Sorry, I'm not a fortune teller. We'll just have to see what happens.'

Such a reply isn't very helpful to the patient, the family, the doctor, or the rest of the health-care team.

It is true that doctors are not very accurate in estimating survival. All too often, doctors make very narrow predictions that turn out to be way off the mark, for example:

'He told me I had 6 weeks to live and I've proved him wrong!'

Despite examples like this, doctors actually tend to overestimate prognosis, and are usually out by a factor of two or more. Experienced clinicians are more accurate than inexperienced ones, but still are only moderately accurate. Despite the deficiencies of clinical estimates, doctors should still attempt to predict the patient's survival as accurately as possible. Such an estimate may still be of use:

- because it enables the clinician to advise the patient and family and to plan care;
- to ensure that the right patients get the right access to services for the terminally ill;
- to determine eligibility for clinical trials.

While it will never be possible to give a precise answer to this question in individual cases, there is a growing literature to indicate that clinical factors can be used to identify a meaningful time range within which the patient's death is likely to occur.

In formulating a response to this question, it is important to be aware that words like prognosis and survival are ambiguous, depending on whether they are being used to refer to diseases (general sense) or individual patients (specific sense). Which sense is appropriate depends on whether the patient has localized cancer, newly identified metastases, or far advanced disease. In newly diagnosed patients with localized cancer who are otherwise well cure may be possible, and the issue of the time of death is irrelevant. Even if cure is not possible, such patients are likely to receive disease-controlling treatment and 5 and 10-year survival rates for the disease are more appropriate than an estimate of individual survival.

In patients with newly-diagnosed metastatic disease, population statistics based on factors such as primary site, sites and extent of metastases, and types of treatment are usually still appropriate. Because survival is less than 12 months in many cases, specific individual factors begin to become important. In patients with far advanced disease, disease-related factors become much less important than specific individual factors.

In patients with far-advanced cancer, such as our patient here, various predictors of survival have been evaluated. They include physiological, pathological, biochemical, clinical, and psychosocial ones. As a result of this research, a pattern has begun to emerge in recent years. Certain laboratory parameters have been found to be associated with a poor survival in patients with advanced cancer. These include high leucocyte count, lymphopaenia, hyperbilirubinaemia, hypercalcaemia, and low acid glycoproteins (reflecting poor hepatic synthesis). When these data are combined with clinical factors, prognostic accuracy is improved.

The performance status of the patient is very important. The Karnofsky Performance Scale score (KPS) correlates closely with survival, but how accurately it predicts the time of death is influenced by the stage of the disease. Even in patients being actively treated, those with a poor performance status (KPS <50) rarely live longer than 6 months. A good performance status does not predict for a long survival in this group, however. The KPS score tends to fall away in the last few weeks of life. One problem with using the KPS is that low scores are dependent on hospitalization as a criterion. As health care delivery changes and sicker patients are cared for at home with increased community support, such definitions become meaningless. A modification of KPS called the PPS (Palliative Performance Status) has been devised recently, although its reliability and validity remains to be tested.

Patients with poor performance status and multiple symptoms do worse than those who are asymptomatic, especially if the symptoms relate to cancer cachexia (anorexia, lack of energy, weight loss). The presence or absence of pain does not seem to be related to survival. In patients with far-advanced cancer, performance status seems to distinguish between those who will live some months and those who will only last days. Although some studies have found 'quality of life' (QOL) scores correlate with survival, others have not. This discrepancy may reflect the domains of QOL that a particular questionnaire measures.

In the case of our patient here, you need to enquire about his performance status. If he is spending most of the day in bed at home, it is likely (50 per cent chance) he will die within the next 2 months, and very unlikely (<10 per cent chance), he will still be alive in 9 months time. An answer along the lines of 'you'll probably make it to Easter but probably won't be here for Christmas' will be the most appropriate. Whether or not you decide to tell him this estimation is another matter!

13.3 A patient requests euthanasia

You visit a 76-year-old German widow on your daily ward round. She says she feels a burden on her family and can't go on like this any longer. She asks you to give her a lethal injection. The patient was found to have renal cancer 6 years ago. She had a nephrectomy and has remained well since. Over the last 3 to 4 weeks, she has had increasing pain in the right hip, worse on weight bearing. Radiographs show metastases in the right femur. Palliative radiotherapy to the right hip is planned.

How are you going to respond to her request?
The ethical issues that surround a request for euthanasia are complex and largely beyond the scope of a clinical manual. The clinical issues though are simpler and should be addressed largely independently of the ethical aspects. A request for euthanasia is a clinical development that must be evaluated and managed like any other. The clinician must unearth its cause and then initiate an appropriate management plan. Before doing so, it is important to understand that euthanasia is a direct action taken at the request of the patient with the primary intention of immediately ending the patient's life. Such an action needs to be clearly differentiated from the decision to forgo life sustaining treatment, and from the desire expressed by

some terminally ill patients to wish that their lives might soon end naturally. If this distinction is not clear in the mind of the health care professional, a deal of unnecessary confusion and anxiety may occur. The provision of adequate pain relief or other symptom control measures and the removal of unwanted, overly burdensome, life prolonging treatment must never be confused with acts of euthanasia.

A request for euthanasia is always a sign that the patient is in extreme distress. Behind this are a myriad of possible underlying factors that may be contributing to this distress. In ethical debates about euthanasia, it is usually assumed that the patient making the request is competent and has carefully considered all his/her options before the request is made. *In clinical practice this situation is rare.* The clinician's first task is to ascertain whether the patient is truly competent, or whether the request in fact represents the first sign of an illness that would normally rob the patient of competence such as a delirium or major depression. Both conditions are very common in the seriously ill and both are amenable to treatment. In these cases, the requests will usually disappear when the underlying condition is treated. Delirium and depression may also underlie a patient's request for the cessation of active treatment, and clinicians must consider these diagnoses before acting on these requests also.

Even when the patient is technically competent, a request for euthanasia often arises when the patient feels that things are hopeless or that their life is out of control. In this situation the physician should try to discover why it is that the patient feels this way. Contributors often include uncontrolled pain, loss of independence, social isolation, or the feeling that one is a burden. Very often these factors can be addressed and reversed. Pain may be amenable to alternative analgesic therapies. Independence may be enhanced by a change in circumstances. Social isolation may be reversed with simple support and feelings of burden with simple reassurance. Again these issues may also play a role in a request for cessation of active treatment and again the clinician should consider these issues before precipitously complying with such requests.

On occasion, competent patients will make requests for euthanasia or for assistance to die that will not dissipate with symptom control and support. Such patients may have had a philosophical commitment to euthanasia that long predated their current situation. This situation is so uncommon that the physician who is faced with such a scenario would be well advised to seek a second opinion to ensure that some underlying cause has not been missed.

Currently, almost all legal jurisdictions prohibit both euthanasia and physician assisted suicide. Whatever the clinician's personal feelings on these laws, there is little ethical or legal justification for complying with the patient's request. In most jurisdictions, those who do so place themselves at risk of prosecution. Even if such a prosecution were not eventually successful, the stress associated with the judicial process would undoubtedly impair professional functioning and limit the clinician's ability to assist other patients in need. Democracies have established methods whereby those who disagree with the law can attempt to change it. Physicians who feel strongly that euthanasia law should be changed are at liberty to follow these routes and should do so rather than flout existing law because 'they know best'.

Competent patients who persistently request euthanasia must be told that the sort of assistance they desire is the sort of assistance that is beyond the power of the physician to provide. The patient should be reassured that the physician has understood their request and is not angered or disempowered by it. It should be made explicit that the physician's inability to meet this request does not equate to a general powerlessness to provide help and that whatever the coming days hold, the clinician will be there to provide whatever support or comfort they can.

13.4 Dealing with angry patients or carers

With appropriate treatment (radiotherapy to the right hip and increased analgesia) and support from ward staff, the patient's pain improves and she stops asking for euthanasia. She regains her mobility and returns home. A month later she is readmitted with right shoulder pain, shortness of breath, and decreased mobility. She has lost a great deal of weight. On admission she is found to have multiple lung metastases, a metastasis in the right scapula, and mild hypercalcaemia. The analgesics are increased but she remains distressed by pain. You receive a phone call from her son who is very angry. He says that you are making her suffer and wants the morphine dose rapidly escalated.

How will you deal with his criticism?
Anger is a common and normal reaction to bad news, signalling frustration and annoyance when events go contrary to expectations and needs are not met. In the cancer arena, people may react with anger to the knowledge that they have a serious disease which may lead to bodily mutilation and shorten their life. Patients may feel it is unfair that this has happened to them and not others, and that their god (if they are religious) has abandoned them. Loss of control is another common cause of anger, when patients find themselves dependent on others, especially if they have been used to being in a dominant or powerful position. They may feel angry at their own powerlessness to affect the outcome, and angry with themselves if they feel they have contributed through past behaviours to the development of their disease. They may also be angry for specific reasons, such as a late diagnosis, delayed referral, perceived inadequate care, or uncontrolled pain. Importantly, anger may be caused by events quite unrelated to the cancer, such as family problems, but be outwardly directed towards the cancer.

In moderation, anger can be a useful motivator for action and an antidote to depression and hopelessness. However, inappropriate levels of anger, out of proportion to the reasons being disclosed, can lead to verbal and even physical abuse of those around them, and decisions which may later be regretted.

The first step in defusing an angry interaction is for the doctor to let the person know in a non-judgemental way, that he or she recognises the anger. You might say something like:

'I can see that this makes you angry.'

Acknowledge its legitimacy, when appropriate:

'Having your hopes and plans for retirement suddenly taken away must be devastating'

and explore the reasons for it:

'What particular aspect of your situation makes you most angry?'

This will prevent anger from building up and exploding, allow open communication to occur, and possibly lead to the exploration of solutions. While it can be difficult, it is important to avoid interpreting anger as a personal attack, directly challenging the patient's interpretation, criticizing patients for their reaction, or getting caught up in defending yourself or other colleagues.

When someone is angry, it can be quite obvious. In others, anger may be hidden under a highly controlled surface or withdrawal. When acknowledging anger, it is important to pick words with an appropriate level of emotion. For example if the person is red in the face and shouting, a response such as:

'You seem a bit irritated'

may escalate the situation:

'Irritated—I'm not irritated—I'm furious. Don't you try and downplay this situation!'

If the person denies anger, it is useful to try and clarify the situation, so a shared understanding of the patient's feelings can be reached:

'I'm sorry—I must have misunderstood you. Tell me more about how you are feeling.'

Usually, recognition and an opportunity to vent feelings will be enough to defuse the situation. Occasionally patients will continue to focus on the issues which make them feel angry. If a genuine wrong has occurred for which the health professional is responsible, it is important to apologize:

'I am sorry. We did mislay your files, and this has slowed things down for you.'

It can be helpful to then restate the goal of the interview:

'I understand that things have happened which have left you feeling very angry, but our goal now is to decide together the best path forward. We need to concentrate on the available treatment options, and what will suit you best.'

If anger persists, alternative causes should be explored:

'Having to wait half an hour to see the doctor has clearly upset you. Have there been other things going on which made the wait particularly trying today?'

Finally, in the face of escalating anger which is non-responsive to the above strategies, setting limits and, if necessary, withdrawing may be appropriate:

'I can see you are really angry about all the tests you have to have. I can't explain what the tests involve and why we think they are necessary while you are so angry. I suggest we have a break to give you some space, and I'll come back in half an hour.'

Facing an angry person can be upsetting and draining for any health professional, especially if the anger is unexpected, directed at staff and apparently unjustified. While the background and strategies described above can be helpful, it is important for health professionals to acknowledge their feelings at the end of such an interview, and to find ways of debriefing, such as talking to colleagues, doing some exercise, or deliberately relaxing.

13.5 A request for alternative medicine

A 42-year-old businessman presents to the oncology clinic with metastatic pancreatic cancer, having had a Whipple's procedure 9 months ago. He now has liver metastases and is in pain, jaundiced, and is losing weight. He has already tried several unproven 'remedies', is on an extreme diet, and has been attending a New Age healer. You offer him enrolment in a trial of palliative chemotherapy. He tells you that on the Internet he has seen a website for a clinic in Tijuana, Mexico. The website reports cures of pancreatic cancer with laetrile and coffee enemas, without side effects, and without any damaging effects on the immune system. He has been advised by friends who claim to have heard of other patients who were cured at this clinic. His friends also tell him that the medical profession has a closed mind to the potential values of such therapies. He plans to sell the family house and fly to Tijuana for the treatment.

How will you handle this problem?
Unconventional and alternative therapy is a controversial topic and can provoke angry emotions in rational, science-orientated physicians. Paradoxically, it may be a source of hope for many patients. It is hard to argue against unproven therapies that primarily aim to enhance quality of life, such as exercise, nutrition, and spiritual approaches. However, the physician has a responsibility to be actively involved in discouraging patients from pursuing expensive and dangerous remedies such as that proposed here.

To do this, the physician needs to have a clear understanding of the differences between conventional cancer treatment and unproven 'alternative'

therapies. Conventional treatments are responsible, objective, reproducible, and have been reliably demonstrated to be safe and effective in
controlling or curing cancer. By contrast, alternative therapies have not
been scientifically tested, their advocates believing the scientific method is
not applicable to the evaluation of their therapies, relying instead on
theories and anecdotes. Far from being 'natural' and 'non-toxic', some can
be very damaging, both physically and psychologically, and may often
interfere with administration of orthodox therapies. The practitioners may
be fraudulent and their treatments may impose severe financial burdens.
Therefore, while it is a general duty of the physician to respect the wishes
and values of the patient, he/she also has a responsibility to:

(1) ensure these values are based on accurate information about the disease
    and its possible treatment; and
(2) protect the patient from exploitation, deception, and harm.

The patient appears to understand that you do not think that travelling to Mexico
for treatment is in his interests, but he insists on going ahead. He wants you to
provide him with documentation to expedite his overseas travel.

Are you obliged to co-operate?
This is another complex issue. Certainly doctors are obliged to respect a
patient's right to *refuse* treatment, but when it comes to complying with a
patient's request to *receive* treatment, things are less clear. There is an
undisputed duty of care to meet *reasonable* requests for treatment. Some
types of alternative therapy could conceivably fall under the umbrella of
'reasonable requests' (e.g. meditation, relaxation therapy) but in this case
the proposed therapy is patently against the patient's interests, and we
would suggest that the doctor is in fact obliged *not* to co-operate. Therefore,
he/she should not provide the patient with the requested documentation.

The patient becomes angry when you refuse his request, and threatens to go and
find a doctor who will provide him with what he wants.

How will you respond to this turn of events?
We have already seen how to deal with the angry patient (Case 13.4). In
denying the request, we must be careful to avoid confrontation, which will
help neither party. This patient is terminally ill and very vulnerable. He
needs ready access to a sympathetic physician or surgeon with which to
discuss his latest hope. Not all doctors will be comfortable with this, but
perhaps times are changing.

It seems that many, if not most, cancer patients try some form of alternative therapy or other during their illness. What is the attraction? Clearly it is
the result of many factors:

(1) the public is aware that cancer is frequently not curable with conven-
    tional therapy;

(2) using these therapies allows the patient and family to reduce anxiety and retain a sense of control;

(3) prevailing social and cultural issues such as individual autonomy, consumerism, and a mistrust of authority (including organized health care)

(4) an aggressive action-orientated approach to health care;

(5) New Age spirituality as a response to life-threatening illness.

A cancer diagnosis is a potent source of suffering—defined as the perceived disintegration of the self—because the impact of cancer devastates all levels of an individual's state of existence—molecular, structural, functional, organizational, and social (there are other levels validated by shared experience: spiritual, artistic, creative). That patients seek alternative therapists and their remedies suggests that conventional treatment is perceived as being unable to meet one or more of these needs. Practitioners of scientific medicine should not be frustrated at the lack of success in areas of the human condition that fall outside the biomedical domain. Rather, we need to acknowledge that patients with cancer have psychosocial and spiritual needs as well as physical ones and that a multidimensional, patient-centred approach to cancer care is required. Strategies for fostering and maintaining hope, even in the face of progressive disease, can be developed by the conventional health-care team. These may ultimately serve the patient's interests far better than alternative medicine.

13.6 'Not for resuscitation' orders

You are the physician on service in a community hospital. A 46-year-old woman with end-stage metastatic melanoma is brought by her family to the emergency department because she has abdominal pain and shortness of breath. She is too weak to walk to the bathroom and they can no longer manage her care at home. She has received all her treatment in the cancer centre of the university teaching hospital 50 kilometres away and you have not met her or her family before. She is cachectic and is clearly dying and needs to be admitted to hospital.

The nursing staff asks you whether you are going to withhold cardiopulmonary resuscitation (CPR) or not.

What should you do?

The patient should be documented **'Not for CPR'**.

It is the doctor's legal responsibility to act in this way, in the patient's best interests. It is controversial, however, as to whether the decision to withhold resuscitation needs to be discussed with the patient and/or the family, or not.

As with other clinical decision making in the context of advanced disease, the decision to withhold CPR depends on: the scientific facts of the case; the burdens, risks, and benefits of the proposed intervention; the patient/family's goals, priorities, and expectations; the patient's rehabilitation potential; ethical and legal issues. There are two main reasons for deciding to withhold CPR in this case, the scientific facts and the ethical/legal context.

Firstly, CPR in patients with advanced malignancy is very rarely successful. The chance of patients with metastatic cancer surviving to discharge home after in-hospital CPR has been estimated to be about 1 per cent, and in one American study almost 90 per cent of physicians felt that CPR should not be performed routinely in patients with widespread cancer. The small chance of benefit is far outweighed by the potential burdens involved.

Secondly, CPR is a medical intervention designed to restore circulation in the event of a cardiac arrest. It is intended to be used in patients who are expected to return to normal functioning, or at least regain a reasonable level of function after the condition that caused the arrest is reversed. It is not intended to prevent dying in patients who are terminally ill. In the context of a terminal illness, such as in this patient's case where death is anticipated, CPR is not justifiable and a 'not for CPR' order is ethically justified.

The process of making the decision is just as important as the decision itself, and this is where the controversy arises. Whether or not the decision should be discussed with the patient is disputed, and depends on whether it is thought that the patient's/family's consent is required. Certainly where the outcome of a CPR intervention is uncertain (e.g. a young patient with good performance status receiving the first cycle of palliative chemotherapy for metastatic cancer who becomes septic from febrile neutropaenia), anticipatory discussions should be held and should cover the extent of resuscitation facilities available, the likelihood of success, and the resulting quality of life. Time taken to discuss these issues should not be a major consideration as most NFR orders can be obtained within 15 min. Many would argue that even if the patient is terminally ill and CPR would almost certainly be unsuccessful, the decision to withhold treatment should normally be discussed with the patient if they are competent to do so, as the doctor–patient relationship should be based on openness, truthfulness, and trust. Many terminally ill patients like to discuss the decision even if most of them leave it up to the doctor to decide. On the other hand, it is argued that there is no obligation for a doctor to discuss with patients futile treatments that will not be offered, as raising such issues is redundant and potentially distressing, undermining rather than increasing autonomy.

There is no legal requirement to discuss resuscitation with the family unless they are appointed as the decision-maker through the Guardianship Board or an enduring power of attorney. However, in the context of terminal illness, where the patient and family are considered the 'unit of care', discussion of such decisions may be important in maintaining the caring relationship.

The decision should also be discussed with members of the multidisciplinary team and clearly documented in the case notes, as well as the concurrent comfort care needs of the patient.

13.7 Managing the last 48 hours of life

A few days later, the patient has been unable to take anything by mouth for several days. You commenced her on a subcutaneous infusion of morphine and haloperidol. Despite this, she is moaning and has myoclonic jerking. The team has ceased all her oral medications, which had included diclofenac, chlotride, and laxatives.

What issues would you consider in her management now?
After assessing the patient and before instigating a management plan, it is vital to spend some time with the family and significant others, assessing their level of understanding of the extent of the patient's cancer, their level of acceptance of the futility of further anticancer therapy or any lifeprolonging treatments, and their understanding of the imminence of death. The treatment plan should be explained to ensure that they are comfortable with what is being done, including the fact that further hydration or feeding is not being considered and that this will not shorten life.

Moaning in the face of decreased level of consciousness is most likely due to bone pain as her non-steroidal medication has been ceased and it is important to continue this either by the rectal route or using a parenteral non-steroidal by the subcutaneous route. In the face of possible deteriorating renal function, rectal paracetamol could be considered instead. In an unconscious hypercalcaemic patient with prostate cancer, both faecal impaction and urinary retention must be ruled out as a cause of discomfort and moaning.

Myoclonus is reasonably common in the terminal stage and must not be ignored. In this situation it is most likely due to the build up of morphine metabolites in the face of decreasing renal function and the correct management would be to either reduce the dose or increase the time between doses. Other causes of myoclonus to be considered are renal failure, hepatic failure, and hyponatraemia; it can be exacerbated by hypocalcaemia and anticholinergic drugs. If reducing medication results in exacerbation of symptoms, it may be worth using a small dose of a benzodiazepine, such as midazolam or clonazepam, to help reduce the myoclonus.

The next step in managing this patient is to consider what other symptoms may occur and plan the next 24 to 48 hours. There may be increasing agitation in the face of hypercalcaemia requiring subcutaneous haloperidol or chlorpromazine suppositories. These should be made available either as a standing order for nursing staff if required, or as medication in the home if the patient is at home.

Most patients develop some degree of terminal respiratory secretions which will require prophylactic use of anticholinergics such as hyoscine hydrobromide, hyoscine butylbromide, or glycopyrronium bromide. Studies show that these are equipotent but hyoscine hydrobromide is most frequently used because of its sedative effect. It can, however, also have an excitatory effect which may require coadministration of a benzodiazepine.

Finally, it is vital to prepare the family for the death itself. If at home, ensure adequate nursing, medical, and psychosocial support with enough medications available for crisis management. The local medical officer must be available to sign the death certificate. Families should be encouraged to limit family conflict and keep it away from the bedside and to say their goodbyes. It is important to continuously explain what is happening and to reassure families and carers. This is the time to check if help with funeral arrangements is needed and to link in with bereavement supports. Respect of individual cultural and religious needs is paramount.

References

13.1

Professional Education and Training Committee of the New South Wales Cancer Council and the Postgraduate Medical Council of NSW (1998). *How to break bad news: interactional skills training manual.* NSW Cancer Council.

Charlton, R.C. (1992). Breaking bad news. *Medical Journal of Australia*, **157**, 615–621.

Butow, P.N., Maclean, M., Dunn, S.M., *et al.* (1997). The dynamics of change: cancer patients' preferences for information, involvement and support. *Annals of Oncology*, **8**, 857–863.

Dunn, S.M., Butow, P.N., Tattersall, M.H. (1993). General information tapes inhibit recall of the cancer consultation. *Journal of Clinical Oncology*, **11**, 2279–2285.

Mackillop, W.J., Stewart, W.E., Ginsberg, A.D., *et al.* (1988). Cancer patients' perceptions of their disease and its treatment. *British Journal of Cancer*, **58**, 355–358.

13.2

den Daas N. (1995). Estimating the length of survival in end-stage cancer: a review of the literature. *Journal of Pain and Symptom Management*, **10**, 548–55.

Maltoni, M., Nanni, O., Pirovano, M. *et al.* (1999). Successful validation of the Palliative Prognostic Score in terminally ill cancer patients. *Journal of Pain and Symptom Management*, **17**, 240–247.

Anderson, F., Downing, G.M., Hill, J., *et al.* (1996). Palliative Performance Scale (PPS): a new tool. *Journal of Palliative Care*, **12**, 5–11.

13.3

Glover, J. (1977). *Causing death and saving lives.* Penguin: London.

Ashby, M. (1997). The fallacies of death causation in palliative care. *Medical Journal of Australia*, **166**, 176–77.

van der Weyden, M.B. (1997). Deaths, dying and the euthanasia debate in Australia. *Medical Journal of Australia*, **166**, 173–4.

13.4

Faulkner, A., Maguire, P., and Regnard, C. (1994). Dealing with anger in a patient or relative: a flow diagram. *Palliative Medicine*, **8**, 51–57.

Kissane, D.W. (1994). Managing anger in palliative care. *Australian Family Physician*, **23**, 1257–1259.

13.5

Angell, M. and Kassirer, J.P. (1998). Alternative medicine—the risks of untested and unregulated remedies. *New England Journal of Medicine*, **339**, 839–41.

Fletcher, D.M. (1992). Unconventional cancer treatments: professional, legal and ethical issues. *Oncology Nursing Forum*, **19**, 1351–4.

Durant, J.R. (1998). Alternative medicine: an attractive nuisance (edit.). *Journal of Clinical Oncology*, **16**, 1–2.

13.6

Miller, D.L., Gorbien, M.J., Simbartl, L.A. *et al.* (1993). Factors influencing physicians in recommending in-hospital pulmonary resuscitation. *Archives of Internal Medicine*, **153**, 1999–2003.

Bruce-Jones, P.N. (1996). Resuscitation decisions in the elderly: a discussion of current thinking. *Journal of Medical Ethics*, **22**, 286–91.

Joint Ethics Working Party, National Council for Hospice and Specialist Palliative Care Services and the Association for Palliative Medicine of Great Britain and Ireland. (1997). CPR for people who are terminally ill. *European Journal of Palliative Care*, **4**, 125.

13.7

Hughes, A., Wilcock, R., Corcoran, R., Lucas, V., and King, A. Audit of clinical guidelines and use of anticholinergic drugs for managing retained secretions in the terminal phase. Free paper, Fifth Congress of the European Association for Palliative Care.

Weatherall, D.J., Ledingham, J.G.G., and Warrell, D.A. (eds) (1992). *Oxford textbook of medicine* (3rd edn). Oxford University Press.

Index